# Seeing the Light

To Esther,
With warmest
regards,
Sharon Gottlieb.

# Seeing the Light

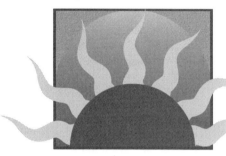

## Eat Well, Be Active, Feel Good About Yourself, Once and For All

*Sharon Gottlieb, RD*

The Nutrition Institute

The information in this book is for reference and education purposes only. It is not intended to be a substitute or replacement for the advice of a physician, dietitian or related health professional. The publisher and the author specifically disclaim any liability, loss, or risk that is incurred as a consequence, directly or indirectly, of the use or application of any of the contents of this book. Consult your physician before making changes to your dietary habits and before starting an exercise program.

Nutrition analysis of the recipes was completed using the nutritional analysis software, Nutritionist IV, Version 3.0, N-Squared Computing, San Bruno, California, supplemented when necessary by information from reliable sources. The nutrition analysis information is provided as an approximate guide to the nutritional composition of the recipes with respect to total energy, fat, carbohydrate and protein content. Actual values can vary depending upon products used, cooking methods and times. Optional ingredients, garnishes and accompaniments were not included in the analysis.

**Canadian Cataloguing in Publication Data**

Gottlieb, Sharon
    Seeing the Light : eat well, be active, feel good about yourself, once and for all
Includes index.
ISBN 0-9685742-0-3

1. Weight loss.   2. Low-calorie diet.   3. Nutrition.   I. Title.
RA784.G68 1999    613.2'5    C99-901008-5


Book Design, Page Composition: Steve Eby
Printer: Transcontinental Printing Inc.
Author Photograph: Keith Penner

Published in Canada by
The Nutrition Institute
60 East Beaver Creek Road
Richmond Hill, Ontario
L4B 3L1

www.seeingthelight.com

Printed and bound in Canada

*To Norman,*

my partner in life, who makes me laugh
and helps make my dreams come true.

# Contents

# Foreward

Sharon was one of the most enthusiastic students I have taught in over 25 years as a Professor of Nutrition. The commitment, curiosity and cooperative nature she brought to her studies have been transformed into a professional approach that works.

Her personal experience and insight, coupled with the expertise of a professional have helped many clients. In one book she has captured the essence of her successful practice to work for a wider audience. Her advice is worthy, practical and effective. Follow this advice and you will be the winner of a healthier lifestyle and a more positive self-esteem.

Sharon knows her business. First she lived it; then she studied it; now she shares it with anyone willing to follow her guidance to seeing the light.

Bon appetit, bonne chance.

DR. RENA MENDELSON
Associate Vice-President, Academic,
Ryerson Polytechnic University

# Sharon's clients say...

"For an encouraging and liveable approach to weight and a healthy sense of self, Sharon's approach is a delight! She offers not only an informed understanding of human needs and foibles when it comes to food, but the support to shift easily to a style of selecting, cooking and eating food that is as painless as any change can be. Read her book and be a collaborator in a gratifying venture that leads to looking and feeling better for keeps!"

"My life has been an 'eatathon.' With Sharon's guidance, I'm starting to see the light."

"The soup recipes are wonderful. Not only are they filling, tasty and nutritious, they're also a great hit with my family. Two of my favorites are the Gazpacho and the California Vegetable Soup."

"I've dropped 45 pounds and I've kept my weight down. Thank you Sharon, for teaching me a healthy way of living."

"Sharon Gottlieb is a nutrition wise girl with an upbeat approach to healthy eating habits. Sharon shares recipes and ideas that help you embrace a healthy lifestyle. Her motivational skills are accompanied by a sincere commitment to promote well-being."

"Sharon is a knowledgeable, caring motivator with expertise on healthy eating. With Sharon's help, one can embrace success, enjoy new ideas while taking positive steps toward a healthy lifestyle.'

"Sharon helps me keep focused on a positive approach to healthy eating and living."

"I have never followed an eating plan that is easier. I feel good about myself, I have reduced my weight and I have never felt better. This is the way I will eat for the rest of my life because it is the only way to eat."

# Acknowledgements

There are countless people who have helped make this book possible. I would like to acknowledge them here, in case I have been remiss in not thanking them in person for their invaluable help, inspiration and support.

First and foremost, I would like to express my heartfelt appreciation to my loving family who have been unwavering in their support of all my professional endeavors and activities.

I am also sincerely indebted to: Dr. Rena Mendelson, the faculty at Ryerson Polytechnic University, and the dietitians at St. Michael's Hospital, who, as outstanding educators, prepared me to be the nutrition professional that I am today; my dear friend, Myrna Riback who has been a caring muse and skillful editor; Linda Barnard for her help with the early editing and for adding some light touches to the manuscript; Steve Eby for his patience with me and for his creative flare in designing the cover, the look of the book and the layout of the pages; Margaret Condy for her assistance with the indexing; Judi Lee-McKee of Transcontinental Printing for her enthusiastic help with this project.

I also want to acknowledge John Wildman, President, the staff and the members of The Fitness Institute, for believing in me and for their positive influence on my personal and professional life.

Finally, I would like to thank the wonderful clients that I have the privilege of working with every day. You inspire and motivate me more than you know. You allow me to share in your success and make not only yourselves, but me, look and feel good in the process.

I thank you all.

SHARON GOTTLIEB

**light n.** the natural agent that stimulates sight and makes things visible; medium or condition of space in which this is present; appearance of brightness; source of light; aspect in which thing is viewed; mental illumination, elucidation; vivacity, enthusiasm, or inspiration in person's face, esp. in eyes; one's mental powers; eminent person; bright parts of picture etc.; window or opening in wall to let light in; (in crossword etc.) word to be deduced from clues.

**light a.** not heavy, easy to lift; (of food) easy to digest; easily borne or done; free from sorrow, cheerful.

Adapted from *The Oxford Dictionary of Current English*, Oxford University Press, Oxford, 1989.

# PART 1

# *Seeing is Believing*

*T*HIS BOOK IS ABOUT seeing and believing that you can eat well, be active, feel good about yourself, once and for all. It's the book I wish I'd had when I was struggling with my own weight, food and eating problems. When I became a dietitian, I vowed I would write it for those who would follow on their journey toward living life in a healthy way.

As you read these words, you may be be thinking that the road ahead looks long. I know how you feel. I know because I've been where you might be right now.

This book is for all the women, teens and men who are facing personal challenges as they try to achieve a healthier lifestyle. Many women like myself have had to struggle with years of dieting and feeling like a failure. A growing number of teens are dealing with self-esteem issues like I did as a result of growing up overweight in a thin-coveting world. Men have their hurdles too. Maybe their doctor has told them they need to reduce their high blood pressure or cholesterol. Or they've come to the conclusion on their own that it's time to get moving and do something about their expanding waistlines. Changing aspects of your life, no matter who you are, is never easy.

> *This book is for all the women, teens and men who are facing personal challenges as they try to achieve a healthier lifestyle.*

## My Story

Let me start by telling you about my own struggle with weight and body image. I grew up as an overweight child. By the time I was eight or ten years old, I was on my first of many diets. I was just a little girl, but I was on a diet.

Of course my family had the best of intentions in trying to help me reduce my weight. Those of you who have overweight children know that you would do almost anything to help them shed those extra pounds and be like all the other kids. And those of you who were like me, overweight as youngsters, I don't have to tell you how cruel kids can be to their pals with a few extra pounds.

No matter how hard I tried, nothing seemed to help. The more my food portions were weighed and measured for me, the more overweight I seemed to grow. The truth was I had become a sneak eater. I ate very properly when everyone was watching. But when I was alone, look out. I ate everything in sight! As much as I covered my tracks, the results of my sneak eating were plain to see, right there on my body.

As I look back, I understand now the reason for my sneak eating. I was truly hungry. Not just for food, but for the emotional comfort I craved for the shame, low self-esteem and feelings of failure I felt for being overweight in a thin-obsessed world.

I certainly didn't know how to handle these powerful emotions. So I stuffed them down with the cookies, crackers and chocolates I devoured when no one was watching. The more sneak eating I did, the more guilt and failure I felt. Of course, this led to more sneak eating and on it went. It was a devastating cycle and I didn't know how to stop.

I tried a number of diets throughout my teens, but my first real "success" with reducing my weight came when I was twenty years old. I joined something new, a diet club. I put the word success in quotation marks, because if you measure success with pounds lost, I guess I was a winner. I lost twenty-five pounds and even received a pin to celebrate my accomplishment. Little did I know I had just climbed aboard the diet roller-coaster and I was in for a long ride.

You see, I was now a committed dieter. When I was "good" on my diet, I chose only low calorie foods. When I was "bad", I'd "cheat" and I was "out of control". To me, dieting became a natural way of eating, typical for many like myself who grew

*Little did I know I had just climbed aboard the diet roller-coaster and I was in for a long ride.*

up on a diet of dieting. But when it came to healthy eating, I didn't have a clue.

Today in my nutrition practice, my clients and I never use what I call "diet talk" when describing how and what we eat. How can anyone feel good about themselves when they say they're "bad", they've "cheated" and they're "out of control"? These are words for criminals, not for someone whose only indiscretion might be to enjoy a favorite dessert or an extra helping of food.

My chronic dieting continued into the early years of my marriage. Thank goodness I was smart enough not to diet when I was pregnant. Liberated from dieting, I went to the other extreme. With each of my three pregnancies my weight climbed to almost two hundred pounds. After I gave birth each time, I started dieting to lose the weight.

And I'd be smoking, after I'd given it up for nine months during my pregnancies for fear of harming my unborn child. But after I gave birth, I'd start again, believing that I needed to smoke to help me shed those pounds. All that mattered was to be slim again. So I'd light up. I'd come a long way, baby!

After the birth of my third child, my husband Norman (you'll hear more about him later) convinced me to try a different approach. Why not give fitness a try? Fortunately, I had given up smoking by then or I would have needed an oxygen tent to get me through my workout. Along with dieting, I started going to The Fitness Institute on a regular basis. I also enrolled in group nutrition classes.

With the help of the club's dietitian, I learned how to eliminate dieting from my life and replace it with healthy eating. For the first time in my life I ate a real sandwich for lunch. Still one of my favorites, it was a satisfying turkey sandwich, layered with lettuce, cucumber and tomato, slathered with Dijon mustard on whole wheat bread. This was a welcome change from my usual ration of melba toast and cottage cheese that left me hungry and vulnerable to four o'clock snack attacks and nightly binge eating.

With my new healthy way of eating, I discovered that my body could be trusted to know when I was hungry or full. This was very new to me. In the past I had always concentrated on being in control, not on being satisfied. I now learned that food was not my enemy. My body was no longer food's weak-willed accomplice ready to betray me with my next mouthful.

Before long, I reached my healthy weight goal which, I am happy to say, I've been able to maintain from that time on. But what's been even more important, I achieved a positive outlook on food and eating. My dieting days were over for good. I had "seen the light".

*My dieting days were over for good. I had "seen the light".*

I couldn't wait to help others see the light too. I was bursting to share what I had learned with everyone who was struggling with their own weight and food issues the way I had.

But I did have to wait a few years because first I wanted to become a Registered Dietitian. It was very important to me to gain the knowledge and professional training that I knew I needed to counsel others.

So with a husband, three young children, and three years experience as an elementary school teacher, I enrolled as a special student at Ryerson Polytechnic University to study food and nutrition.

And did I feel special! As I sat in my first nutrition class, my eyes filled with tears, so overjoyed and enormously grateful was I at how far I'd come. I know this might sound corny, but I felt I was the luckiest person in the world.

In the four years that followed, I studied, interned and graduated. I loved every minute of it. I treasured every morsel of knowledge and bit of experience I gained about food, nutrition and health. Nothing seemed unimportant or irrelevant to me. I soaked up everything like a sponge. And I'm happy to say, four years after I started back to school, I was still at my healthy weight goal and ready to help others achieve their goals too.

After a brief stint as an outpatient dietitian in a teaching hospital, I started my own nutrition consulting practice at The Fitness Institute, the very place that I got my start on a healthier lifestyle. My life had come full circle.

## Seeing is Believing

Which brings me to you. Why am I telling you all this? Because I want you to see that I have been where you might be right now. I know from firsthand experience what works and what doesn't.

What doesn't work is dieting, because all you ever become is a good or bad dieter like I was, knowing very little about healthy eating. What does work is eating delicious, healthy, flavorful foods, being active and feeling good about yourself, once and for all.

And who better to teach you than me, a former overweight, chronic dieter turned professional dietitian, healthy eater? I bet we have a lot in common.

When I was overweight, the heaviest thing about me was not my body. It was my heart. My heart was weighed down with the guilt and shame of being overweight in a society that worshipped thinness. When I saw the light in more ways than one—about what I ate, how I lived and most importantly, how I viewed the whole process, I was truly on the path to achieving and maintaining a healthier lifestyle, once and for all. And so will you.

As I mentioned earlier, my clients and I never use words like "good", "bad" or "cheat" when we talk about food. So you

*When I was overweight, the heaviest thing about me was not my body. It was my heart.*

won't be reading them in this book when it comes to healthy eating. And from now on, we won't be saying "losing" when it comes to weight. You, my friend, are a winner!

It's only in the weight game that winners strive to lose and success is measured by what is lost. So from now on aim to achieve your healthy weight goal, not on losing weight. Give it a try. I guarantee you'll feel better about yourself and what you're doing right away.

Now that we've got that out of the way, let me tell you how this book will work for you. It's really three books in one.

Part One, Seeing is Believing, is your road map. It will provide you with the tips and strategies you're going to need on your way to accomplishing your healthy eating goals. It will help you in those tricky situations like dining at a buffet, watching TV without munching, or dealing with feelings like anger, frustration or boredom without turning to food. It will also show you how to get moving and to enjoy active living every day.

In Part Two, you'll find the Recipes for Success. These fast and easy recipes are delicious, low in fat and light on calories. I know you're going to love them. My clients and members of The Fitness Institute certainly do.

Part Three is your Personal Journal. It's your special place where you can do some planning, write down what you're eating, what you're thinking, how you're feeling and anything else that will help you keep a positive focus as you achieve your goals.

So there you'll have it, along with some of my personal stories and experiences that I want to share with you. Along the way, you're going to learn that you can and will achieve your healthy eating and lifestyle goals, once and for all, as long as you believe in yourself and in what you're doing.

So let's get busy "seeing the light".

*It's only in the weight game that winners strive to lose and success is measured by what is lost.*

# CHAPTER 1

# D-i-e-t is a 4-Letter Word

$\mathcal{D}$IET IS A FOUR-LETTER WORD. You probably didn't expect to hear this from a dietitian. After all, I'm not called a "healthyweightician."

My esteemed colleagues and I do plan and design healthy diets to help clients achieve their weight and nutrition goals. In fact, there is actually nothing wrong with the word "diet". Too bad it's a word that's taken on a negative meaning for many in our society.

What "diet" has come to mean is a temporary way of restrictive eating for the purpose of "losing weight". In fact, the going on and off of diets is a national past-time. It is often referred to as the diet roller-coaster or yoyo dieting. No matter what you call it, it's not a ride you want to be on.

The scenario goes something like this. The dieter follows the diet and "loses" a few pounds. The faster the better. But after the initial drop in weight, feelings of deprivation set in. The dieter goes off the diet. The dieter then ends up finding the "lost" pounds plus a few extra for good measure. The dieter ends up heavier in weight and feeling like a failure. This ultimately leads to feelings of guilt, low self-esteem and an unhealthy outlook on food and eating. With each failure, the dieter feels more and more discouraged. I know I did.

*What "diet" has come to mean is a temporary way of restrictive eating for the purpose of "losing weight".*

## What the Heck

Whether it's the grapefruit or cabbage soup diet, high protein or any other new diet on the best-seller list, what they all have in common is that your "success" depends on the strict adherence to the plan.

The minute a "not allowed" food is eaten, you're finished. You've "cheated", you're "bad", you're "out of control" and you feel guilty. Who wouldn't? After all, you didn't stick to the diet. Bad, bad, bad! You shall be punished by being forced to stand on the scale and see a higher number.

So what do you do? You think, "What the heck. I'm off my diet anyway. I might as well eat something—anything that's not nailed down. Today is a write-off. I'll just start again tomorrow." This is a great way of getting nowhere fast. Because in the dieting game, tomorrow takes a long to come, if it does at all.

Achieving your weight goal with healthy eating is a whole other story. With healthy eating, all foods are allowed, so you don't ever have to go "off" anything.

Great, you're thinking, but how are you ever going achieve a healthy weight by eating everything you want? I'll show you how.

Healthy eating is a continuum. It's about making food choices, not about being perfect. Let's face it, none of us is perfect. So breathe a sigh of relief and start enjoying your food.

*With healthy eating, all foods are allowed, so you don't ever have to go "off" anything.*

## Healthy Eating Continuum

| Lower Fat, Lower Calorie Foods | | Higher Fat, Higher Calorie Foods |
|---|---|---|

This is how the healthy eating continuum works. Most of your choices will be made from the "lower fat foods" end of the scale. Your choices will include whole grain breads, cereals, vegetables and fruits, skim or 1% dairy products, leaner meats, poultry or fish and foods prepared with little or no added fat.

Occasionally, depending on the situation, you might have a higher fat food or consume a larger meal. This doesn't mean you are "off" anything or that you've abandoned your commitment to eat in a healthy way.

What it does mean is that on this particular occasion, you've made choices from the "higher fat" end of the continuum. At your next meal, all you need to do is make choices from the "lower fat" end to balance the extra fat and calories. Your goal of healthy eating hasn't changed, and you got to enjoy a favorite food without "blowing" anything or being "bad". Yes, you can have your cake on occasion and eat it too, and achieve your healthy weight and lifestyle goals.

Compare this to a dieting scenario. You've been "perfect" on your diet for ten days. You haven't deviated once. But it's Mary's birthday at work and everyone's chipped in to buy her a birthday cake. After the candles are blown and the birthday song is sung, the cake is cut and the plates are being passed around. You really don't want everyone to know you're on a diet again, so you take a piece of cake. After all, you've been so "good" all week, a little piece of cake won't hurt. The next thing you know, you've devoured a wedge the size of the Titanic. You start getting that sinking feeling. You feel "guilty" because you've "cheated" on your diet and you've been "bad". So what do you do? You say to yourself, "What the heck. Today's a write-off anyway. I might as well join the gang for beer and chicken wings after work. I'll start again on my diet tomorrow."

The next day comes and you resolve to make up for yesterday's "cheating". So you skip breakfast. But by mid-morning, your blood sugar is dropping like a stone. That donut at the coffee shop is awfully hard to resist. When someone suggests

*Occasionally, depending on the situation, you might have a higher fat food or consume a larger meal.*

burgers and fries for lunch, your tummy starts rumbling. You're so hungry, there's no way that a green salad with lemon juice is going to do the trick. You go along and figure you'll definitely start again tomorrow. That evening, you munch your way through a whole bag of potato chips in front of the TV, wash it down with a can or two of soda pop and go on to the ice cream that's been calling to you from the freezer all week. You've blown your diet anyway, so what the heck. You'll start again on Monday.

Does this sound familiar? It sure does to me. And it probably does to you too if you've ever been on a diet. In fact, it's so common researchers identified this eating pattern several years ago by doing a simple experiment.

> *You've blown your diet anyway, so what the heck. You'll start again on Monday.*

## Of Mice and Men

The experiment involved two groups of subjects. The first group had never dieted. The second group were experienced dieters. For them dieting was a way of life. Guess which group I would have been in?

On the day of the experiment, the non-dieters' group came to the lab. It was lunchtime and they were all hungry. When they arrived, they were offered cake and ice cream and were told to eat as much as they wanted. The quantity of cake and ice cream that they consumed was recorded. Because they were hungry, they ate quite a lot.

The same experiment was conducted with the second group, the dieters. They arrived hungry, were offered the cake and ice cream, were told to eat as much as they wanted. The quantity that they consumed was also recorded. The dieting group ate much less cake and ice cream than the non-dieters.

The same experiment was repeated a week later, but there was a minor change in the routine. Each group still arrived hungry, but before they were offered the cake and ice cream, each person was required to drink a milkshake.

This time, the non-dieting group ate much less cake and ice cream than they had the previous week, probably because they had satisfied some of their hunger by drinking the shake. What do you think happened with the dieters' group?

You guessed it. The dieters' group, after drinking the milkshake, ate much more cake and ice cream than they had the previous week. In fact, after drinking the milkshake, they consumed the most cake and ice cream of the entire experiment.

From the results of this and other similar experiments, researchers have concluded that dieting leads to overeating and bingeing. In the dieters' minds, when they drank the milkshake, they had blown their diets, so "what the heck", they might as well go on and eat the cake and ice cream too.

From years of restricting their eating, the dieters didn't respond to physical feelings of hunger and fullness, but were more influenced by whether they believed they were "on" or "off" their diets. When they were "on" their diets they couldn't be tempted to "cheat" even if they were truly hungry. But when they went "off" their diets by drinking the milkshake, then "what the heck", they might as well indulge.

So what's the lesson here? First, if you do choose to have a higher fat food and you like it, enjoy it. It doesn't mean you're "off" anything. It has no bearing on your decision to eat in a healthy way. It just means that you ate a higher fat food and you'll balance this food with a lighter choice at your next meal.

The notion of good and bad foods no longer exists. In its place is the healthy eating continuum which includes all foods from which you are constantly making choices. With the healthy eating continuum, you can occasionally have your cake and still achieve your healthy weight and lifestyle goals, once and for all.

*The notion of good and bad foods no longer exists.*

## If d-i-e-t is a four-letter word for you too, here's what to do:

1. Never refer to yourself or your food choices as "good" or "bad".

2. If you overeat, or eat something that is higher in fat or calories, don't refer to it as "cheating". "Cheat" is too harsh a word to describe something as innocent as choosing something to eat.

3. Don't feel guilty if you've eaten something that is higher in fat or calories. Instead, balance it with a lighter choice at your next meal or snack.

4. Choose your foods along the healthy eating continuum.

5. Avoid "all or nothing" thinking.

6. Aim for making enjoyable, lighter choices, not perfection.

## 10 Steps to Help You See the Light

1. Believe that you can eat well, be active, and feel good about yourself.

2. Aim for progress, not perfection.

3. Focus on achieving, not losing.

4. Avoid all or nothing thinking.

5. Cook with little or no added fat.

6. Make lighter choices when eating out.

7. Include some form of enjoyable physical activity in your day.

8. If you've been filling up on too many bagels and large servings of pasta, replace some of this starch with vegetables and fruit.

9. Enjoy a "mini-meal" as a snack instead of snack-type food choices.

10. Treat yourself well with non-food rewards.

# CHAPTER 2

# Fat is Fattening

## and So is Eating Too Much Fat-Free Food

LIKE MOST PEOPLE TODAY, you may be thinking that buying foods labelled "fat-free", "low-fat" and "lite" will put you on the fast track to a smaller size. "So why isn't this happening?" you ask.

I'll give you my answer, but first, I need to share with you some very simple basics I learned in biochemistry class. Please bear with me because this chapter contains some very valuable information. It will help you understand what food is made of and what your body does with the food once it passes your lips. No, it doesn't just settle on your hips, at least not right away.

Knowing how your body uses food will help you make enlightened choices about what to eat and what to avoid to help you achieve your healthy eating, weight and lifestyle goals, once and for all.

Now at this point you're probably thinking, "I know what to eat. And I know what not to eat—anything that I like or that tastes good! I don't need more information. I just need a diet cop."

> *It will help you understand what food is made of and what your body does with the food once it passes your lips.*

How many times have dietitians heard this one before? It makes me think that I should have enrolled in the police academy instead of food and nutrition school to do my job. Maybe I should be handing out overeating "tickets" instead of menu plans.

But seriously, seeing the light means working with your body, not against it. When you diet to "lose weight", you ignore what's going on from the neck down. Your body becomes just another thing to control along with your appetite, food intake, calories and fat grams.

*When you diet to "lose weight", you ignore what's going on from the neck down.*

With dieting, all that matters is numbers. Numbers manipulated from the command center, your brain, are all that count. Before you know it, you're obsessed with numbers—how much you weigh, how much you should weigh, how many pounds you've lost or gained, how long it will take to reach your goal, and the calories and fat grams in everything. And don't forget how much water you'll have to drink before you see a smaller number on the scale or before you explode, whichever comes first.

By concentrating on numbers instead of on what's happening in your body, you ignore the fact that your body knows what's best for you, even if you don't think so. When you learn to work with your body, not against it, you'll be on your way to achieving your healthy eating and lifestyle goals, once and for all.

## Food Basics

To the body, food is fuel. This seems obvious, but in our culture, food and eating can mean almost anything. Food can be a source of pleasure, comfort, love and entertainment, and an easy way to deal with almost any emotion from anger to zeal. (What other emotion starts with "z"?)

In any case, food provides the body with energy in the form of calories. If you were a car, food would be your gasoline.

Calories come in the form of protein, fat, and carbohydrate. Alcohol also provides the body with calories.

## Protein-Your Building Blocks

Protein is found in meat, fish, poultry, dairy products and eggs. What some people may not know is protein is also found in grains and vegetables. Protein provides four calories per gram. You won't need to count calories, but you do need to know the relative amount of calories that protein, fat, carbohydrate and alcohol provide.

*What some people may not know is protein is also found in grains and vegetables.*

The body uses protein for building blocks. Protein is used to make things. For example, when you eat a piece of chicken, it is broken down into its component parts called amino acids. These amino acids are used in the body to make new things like skin, hair, tissue, enzymes and antibodies.

The body does use some protein for fuel, but the main function of protein is for building material. When the body uses protein for fuel, a waste product is formed that has to be eliminated. This means you need to drink plenty of water, so that the kidneys can flush the waste out of the body.

When people go on very high protein diets, they seem to drop a lot of weight very quickly. But now that you know that the body flushes out plenty of water along with the waste formed when it uses protein for fuel, you can understand why.

Much of this weight is actually water drawn from the body as the waste is being flushed out through the kidneys. Sure, it shows up on the scale as pounds off, but once water balance is restored, the actual weight reduction is much less.

Also, high intakes of protein have been associated with an increased risk of osteoporosis, a weakening of the bones that can result in fractures. This is another important reason to avoid high protein diets for weight reduction, not to mention the saturated fat and cholesterol that are often found in animal protein foods like steak, eggs and bacon.

But you do need enough protein to provide you with the building blocks for growth and repair of tissues. And including a source of lean protein at each meal is a great way to keep you feeling fuller longer. Protein slows food from being emptied from your stomach and thereby helps sustain blood glucose levels.

*And including a source of lean protein at each meal is a great way to keep you feeling fuller longer.*

## Fat—Your Storing Fuel

Fat is fattening. This means that fat provides nine calories per gram, more than double the calories found in protein and carbohydrate. And the sad truth is, the fat that you eat is similar to the fat on your body. It's relatively easy for your body to convert food fat into body fat.

I refer to fat as your storing fuel because very little energy is needed to change food fat into stored body fat. One hundred calories of excess food fat can end up as 97 calories of stored body fat. If only everything were that easy! But the good news is, fat is also a burning fuel. The key to achieving a healthy weight is to burn more than you store.

Humans can store what seems like an almost unlimited number of calories in fat cells. This used to be a good thing. Humans evolved during a time when food was scarce and energy requirements were high. Stored body fat would provide a ready source of energy when food was in short supply. Those who could store fat were most likely to survive periods of famine. Survival of the fattest, you might say.

On the other hand, those who didn't store fat most likely perished. They burned most of the calories they ate and had little in reserve for leaner times. Believe me, not one supermodel cavewoman would have made it in those days.

This ability to store fat has been passed on to us by our fat-storing, thrifty genes. It ensured our survival as a species. In modern times however, machines do much of the physical work for us. Today, our energy needs are pitifully low and for many, food is relatively cheap and plentiful.

As a result, this survival mechanism appears to be contributing more to health risks like obesity, heart disease and diabetes, than to helping us flourish. And, as a society, if we don't collectively start seeing the light in terms of our intake of total calories and fat, the rate of obesity will continue to grow and grow.

Some sources of dietary fat in North America are butter, margarine, oil, salad dressing, cream, cream cheese, mayonnaise, sauces, gravies, fatty meats, and high-fat dairy products. And don't forget baked goods, nuts, chocolate bars, fried and processed foods. I know you probably think that's all the good stuff. We've all been programmed to think this way. From childhood, every time we were given a "treat" like a chocolate bar or a bag of potato chips, we were taught that high fat foods are special. Being forced to eat our carrots and green beans seemed like punishment. No wonder we have so much trouble making healthy food choices today.

As adults, we need to see the light and unlearn this way of thinking. We must value fresh and healthy foods as the real treats. What could be better than a slice of freshly-baked whole grain bread, a steaming bowl of vegetable soup or a dish of succulent berries crowned with a scoop of frozen yogurt? Let's teach our children to enjoy healthy eating by giving them some real treats too.

*Believe me, not one supermodel cavewoman would have made it in those days.*

## Carbohydrate—Your Burning Fuel

The third component of food is carbohydrate which provides four calories per gram. Carbohydrate is found in bread, cereals, grains, pasta, legumes which are dried peas, beans and lentils, vegetables and fruits, sugar, honey and syrup.

Carbohydrate is your burning fuel. It's your gasoline. It's the main fuel for your working muscles and your brain. Carbohydrate can also be turned into fat if eaten in excess, but less efficiently. Still, one hundred excess calories of carbohydrate can end up as approximately 75 calories of fat on your body. This means that about 25% of the calories from excess carbohydrate is used up in the process of changing carbohydrate to fat.

## Fat-Free Alert!

There is now a tremendous variety of lower fat and fat-free food available at the supermarket. Has this helped us reduce our weight?

Apparently not. The number of overweight people in North America continues to be on the rise, even though overall fat consumption is declining. So, with all the lower fat food, nutrition information, products and recipes, North Americans are still getting fatter. Why? The simple reason is we're probably just eating too much, fat-free food included.

A study was conducted on the impact of fat-free food labelling. In the experiment, identical brands of yogurt were offered to two groups of subjects. The group that was offered the yogurt labelled "fat-free" ate more yogurt than the other group who believed the yogurt was higher in fat. It seems that the term "fat-free" has become a licence to overeat. In a similar experiment, those who ate the yogurt labelled "fat-free" were also more inclined to indulge in a higher fat "treat" later on.

They likely believed that because they had been so "virtuous" in choosing the lighter food, they certainly could afford to splurge.

A fat-free product can be very helpful in achieving your healthy weight goal if the lower fat food is eaten in the same amount as its higher fat original. But if you're tempted to eat the whole box of low-fat cookies or munch your way through an entire bag of fat-free pretzels or potato chips, all those extra calories will contribute to weight gain not a lower weight. Fat is fattening, but so is eating too much fat-free food. Remember, a calorie is a calorie. And calories still count.

In the same way, watch out for that word we all love— free. Fat-free doesn't mean calorie-free. Far from it. When fat is removed from a product, fillers and sugars are often added to achieve a desired consistency or to improve taste. These do add calories so that the actual savings in calories may not be very much. A fat-free cookie can have almost as many calories as its higher fat cousin.

*A fat-free cookie can have almost as many calories as its higher fat cousin.*

So the bottom line is, you can substitute fat-free and lower fat products for their higher fat originals, but be aware of portion size to reap the real benefits of eating reduced fat foods. And don't be tempted to reward yourself with higher fat "treats" because you've made the lighter choice.

## Alcohol Equals Empty Calories

Alcohol is found in wine, beer, spirits and liquor. It provides seven calories per gram. These are generally empty calories. This means that they do not provide significant amounts of vitamins or minerals for your body to use. But it's not all bad news. Studies have shown that a moderate intake of alcohol is associated with some health benefits.

A moderate intake of alcohol for women is about four to seven drinks per week. For men it's about one or two drinks per day, a drink being equivalent to 5 ounces/150 mL of wine, 12 ounces/350 mL of beer or 1½ ounces/50 mL of liquor. Beware of sugary mixers. The extra calories they provide add up very quickly.

## The Bottom Line

When we compare protein, fat, carbohydrate and alcohol, it's clear that the two which provide the greatest number of calories are fat and alcohol. I won't dwell on the alcohol issue because it's a personal choice. I'll just say once more that it's recommended that you keep your consumption to no more than four to seven drinks per week for women, and one to two drinks per day for men, unless you choose not to drink at all or your doctor has advised you to avoid alcohol completely.

For those who enjoy an occasional drink, you can still achieve your healthy weight and lifestyle goals without giving up the one beer, glass of wine, or cocktail that you enjoy and may have some benefits.

## How to Stop Storing Fat

Because fat is fattening and fat is your storing fuel, the first step in achieving and maintaining your healthy weight goal is to reduce your intake of fat. Remember, you want to stop being a fat storer.

To do this you first have to reduce the amount of fat you eat. And I'm sure you can list as many low-fat tips as I can because you can't go anywhere these days without hearing the low-fat tune. But knowing what to do and doing it are two different things.

So, to make it happen, start with simple moves like replacing butter and margarine with fruit spread on toast, use oil minimally in stir-fries and salad dressings (always

*But knowing what to do and doing it are two different things.*

measure) and avoid fried foods. These are key strategies to reducing your fat intake without making radical changes that are hard to stick to.

Frying food absorbs a lot of fat, so bake, roast, steam, poach, broil, BBQ or microwave instead. Always have salad dressing served on the side so that you can take a little on your fork to drizzle over your greens. Yes, I said fork, not spoon. Most of the dressing will fall through the tines of the fork. And what's left on the fork can be used to spear your next mouthful. You'll end up eating less dressing and less fat. You'll be amazed at how you won't miss it. Soon, you'll find the thought of a salad swimming in dressing off-putting, to say the least. Or avoid dressing altogether and go for a squeeze of lemon or a dash of a flavorful vinegar like balsamic, wine or rice vinegar.

Instead of cream in your coffee, switch to milk. If you can't bear the look and taste of skim milk in your coffee, reduce the fat step by step. Go from cream to homo, from homo to 2%, from 2% to 1%, and finally to skim. Or try evaporated skim milk which is thicker. By the time you get to skim, cream will taste greasy to you, for sure.

## From Great to Grease to Gross

In my food science course, I learned that fat creates something called a coated mouth-feel. Sounds gross, but believe it or not, that's the sensation people often crave. Those who are used to the coated mouth-feel of fat describe it as creamy, smooth, rich and luxurious. But when they switch to lower fat foods, they soon become unused to it.

If they accidentally pour cream in their coffee instead of milk, they find it feels greasy. Since most people do not love grease, their old favorites lose most of their charm. I've heard

*In my food science course, I learned that fat creates something called a coated mouth-feel.*

this over and over again when my clients have "treated" themselves to fries or chips and end up finding them too oily. When you get to this stage, you'll be well on your way to reaching your healthy eating goals, once and for all.

## Get "Lite" Right

*To get the real benefit, as I've mentioned earlier, use these lighter foods in the portions (or less) than you would their higher fat originals.*

Choose "lite" products to reduce your fat intake whenever possible. This means the light or ultra-light version of mayonnaise, margarine, salad dressing, cream cheese, peanut butter and sour cream. And to get the real benefit, as I've mentioned earlier, use these lighter foods in the portions (or less) than you would their higher fat originals.

For example, don't pour on gobs of salad dressing just because it's "lite". The calories will add up very quickly. Remember, fat is fattening, but so is eating too much fat-free food.

Also, be careful with the term "lite". It can mean light in fat and calories. But as with "lite" olive oil, it can also mean light in color or flavor. So be sure to read the label to make sure "lite" refers to the fat or calorie content, not other things like color, flavor, and texture.

## The Good, the Bad and the Healthy

We've been talking about fat generally, but there are actually three types of dietary fat. Saturated fat is solid at room temperature and is found in foods of animal origin like dairy products other than skim, lard, meats, poultry skin, and in tropical oils such as palm, palm kernel and coconut oil. Saturated fat is the one that raises serum or blood cholesterol.

Polyunsaturated fat is found mainly in vegetable oils like corn, safflower, sunflower and soybean. These provide essential fatty acids. It is believed that small amounts of polyunsaturated fats may help to lower serum cholesterol.

Monounsaturated fat is found in olive, canola and peanut oil. Small amounts of monounsaturated fat may also help to reduce serum cholesterol. Some believe it may be more beneficial in this regard than polyunsaturated fat because it has little effect on lowering HDL, which is the good cholesterol.

A fourth fat, "trans" fat is created in a process called hydrogenation. This changes liquid oil to a solid or semi-solid state so that it can be used in baking, frying or as a spread. Trans fat is found in many processed foods like cookies, crackers, French fries, potato chips and in some margarines. It is believed that trans fat also plays a role in raising serum cholesterol.

## Figuring the Fat

I'd like to focus a little more attention on trans fat. Since a lot of it is consumed in North America, you should know what you're getting if you eat this type of fat.

At the present time, nutrition labels tell you only the amount of total fat and the amount of saturated, polyunsaturated and monounsaturated fat when the fat information is provided. The amount of trans fat contained in the food is not shown even though it may have a similar effect as saturated fat in raising serum cholesterol.

If the list of ingredients on a food package mentions the words "hydrogenated" or "shortening", you can bet there'll be some trans fat hiding somewhere. To see if we're right, let's be a trans fat detective. We can add up the three types of fat on the nutrition information panel on a snack food like potato chips. If the total we get isn't the same as the total fat listed, the missing fat is likely to contain some "trans" fat, which doesn't have to be identified.

*The amount of trans fat contained in the food is not shown even though it may have a similar effect as saturated fat in raising serum cholesterol.*

## Potato Chips (28 g serving)

| | | |
|---|---|---|
| Energy: | 150 calories | |
| Fat: | 10 g | |
| | polyunsaturated fat | 0.4 g |
| | monounsaturated fat | 2.4 g |
| | saturated fat | 1.9 g |
| | | 4.7 g |

10g fat - 4.7g (poly + mono + sat) = 5.3 g unidentified fat

In this food, the amount of fat that can potentially raise cholesterol is really 1.9 grams saturated fat plus the trans fat which can be part of or most of the unidentified fat. This can add up to considerably more than the seemingly low 1.9 grams of saturated fat alone.

Now let's use what I call the "figure the fat" formula to see what percentage of calories is coming from fat in this typical snack food.

Fat (per serving) 10g x 9 calories per gram = 90 calories coming from fat

90 calories from fat divided by 150 calories per serving

= .60 x 100% = 60% of calories coming from fat

It is recommended that we aim for no more than 30% of calories from fat or less. Even though all foods can't fall into the 30% fat or less category, these typical potato chips could put you over the top very easily. And a 28 g (1 oz) serving size? Who eats just 28 g (1 oz) at a sitting?

# The "Lowdown" on Cholesterol

Blood (serum) cholesterol is a fatty, wax-like substance that is manufactured mainly in the liver. It is carried in the bloodstream to all parts of the body. It is a component of cell walls, it is used to produce bile acids which help to digest fat, and to make some hormones and vitamin D.

The production of cholesterol is influenced by genetic and dietary factors. There are two main types of blood (serum) cholesterol. HDL (high density lipoprotein), is the "good" or "healthy" cholesterol because it gathers up excess cholesterol in the bloodstream and carries it back to the liver to be used or excreted by the body. It's like a cholesterol-hungry scavenger that gobbles up the excess in your blood.

*The production of cholesterol is influenced by genetic and dietary factors.*

Then there's LDL (low density lipoprotein). It's the "bad" cholesterol because this is the one that can build up in the arteries. An elevated level of serum cholesterol is associated with an increased risk of atherosclerosis. When there is too much cholesterol in the bloodstream, it can settle on the inside of artery walls. This can cause arteries to become clogged and increase the risk of heart attack or stroke.

The cholesterol that is found in foods is called "dietary" cholesterol. It can affect serum cholesterol to some extent, but the amount and type of fat consumed are far more significant. Dietary cholesterol is found in animal foods like dairy products, meats, poultry, and fish, egg yolks, organ meats, shrimp and caviar. Why did I emphasize animal foods? Because only animals have livers, and livers make cholesterol.

Now back to our potato chips. Until recently, potato chips were marketed as a "cholesterol-free" snack food. We all know that a potato doesn't have a liver. Nor does vegetable oil, hydrogenated or otherwise. So the "cholesterol-free" claim was virtually meaningless, especially in light of the high total fat and the potentially cholesterol-raising trans and saturated fat combo. Be sure to look beyond "cholesterol-free" and other claims when evaluating the health benefits of the foods you choose.

You can practise being a trans fat detective and figuring the fat in Part 3, Personal Journal.

## Calorie-Wise, Fat is Fat

When it comes to dietary fat, it is important to remember that all fats provide nine calories per gram and all are potentially fattening. This means that whether it's heart-healthy olive oil or potentially artery-clogging lard, fat is fattening. When it comes to fat, consume small amounts and be sure to choose the healthy ones when you do.

## Have Your Meat and Heart Health Too (or "She Loves You, Yaa, Yaa, Yaa")

I'll let you in on four tips that will allow you to enjoy any type of meat, fish or poultry your healthy heart desires. I call them the Fab Four, in honor of John, Paul, George and Ringo. I was always a Beatles fan. I even went to a live concert when I was fourteen years old. I couldn't hear for a week for all the music and the noise. I lost my voice for all the screaming and the crying we did at seeing our idols. But it was worth it! So will following the Fab Four when it comes to enjoying meat, fish and poultry.

**Fab 1:** eat these high protein foods lean and well-trimmed of all visible fat. Avoid chicken skin and wings which contain most of the fat in poultry. Forget about the deep-fried chicken wings. They're a fat double whammy. Trim all visible fat from meats before cooking and eating.

**Fab 2:** prepare meat, fish and poultry using a low-fat cooking method like broiling, roasting, baking, poaching, microwaving, BBQing, and stir-frying with little or no added fat.

**Fab 3:** consume about six ounces (175 g) of cooked, lean protein food per day. I know this doesn't sound like very much. But if you recall what I said earlier, your body doesn't run on protein. Protein is not a major source of fuel.

To go to work, drive carpool, work on your computer, play squash, do housework, mow the lawn, and talk on the phone, you're using very little protein for fuel. You're mostly using a combination of carbohydrate and fat. So you don't need to overeat on protein. And by eating a moderate amount of protein you'll automatically reduce your fat intake, especially saturated fat.

Generally, a well-balanced diet, with choices from all four food groups will provide a healthy adult with all the protein he or she needs.

**Fab 4:** variety. This happens to be one of the most important basics of healthy eating. Choose a variety of protein foods and you'll be able to enjoy them all. Let me show you how.

*Choose a variety of protein foods and you'll be able to enjoy them all.*

A week's worth of supper entrées might include: a portion of grilled lean beef, about the size of the palm of your hand or a deck of cards; a chicken and vegetable stir-fry made with a minimum of oil; vegetarian chili; a broiled veal burger; baked haddock; tofu lasagna; and an egg white frittata.

See what I mean? You don't have to eat a skinless chicken breast every night of the week until you're ready to cluck, to eat in a healthy way. Just remember the Fab Four when it comes to eating protein foods.

**Fab 1:** lean and well-trimmed

**Fab 2:** a low-fat cooking method

**Fab 3:** the equivalent of six ounces cooked protein per day

**Fab 4:** variety

## Don't Give Up on Dairy

People often ask me if they should give up dairy foods to achieve their weight and health goals. They'd heard that all dairy products were high in fat and they would get better results by eliminating dairy products completely. Wrong on both counts.

In fact, the exact opposite is true. Skim milk and nonfat yogurt are virtually fat-free and certainly should be part of a healthy eating plan. When choosing milk, yogurt and cottage cheese, look for 1% milkfat or less.

Hard cheeses like cheddar and Swiss are another story. They're generally high in fat. Typically, cheddar cheese is about 34% milkfat by weight but it actually derives about 75% of its calories from fat. A part-skim cheese, with 15% milkfat, derives about 50% of its calories from fat and a 7% milkfat cheese, still gets about 33% of its calories from fat.

So to keep fat intake low, consume cheese in small amounts, perhaps as an ingredient in a low-fat veggie lasagna, pizza or pasta dish, but not as an everyday sandwich filling or snack.

Although not a dairy product, you might be wondering if you should be eating eggs. The egg was once considered the "gold" standard of protein food. In recent years, eggs have lost some of their luster because of their relatively high cholesterol content.

The bad news about eggs is that the yolk contains about 200 mg of cholesterol. If you're trying to lower serum cholesterol, you should follow a low-fat diet and consume no more than 300 mg of dietary cholesterol per day. One egg yolk con-

*In recent years, eggs have lost some of their luster because of their relatively high cholesterol content.*

tains about two-thirds of your daily quota. Also, the yolk contains about 5 grams of fat. That's the amount of fat in one teaspoon of oil.

The good news about eggs though, from a fat and cholesterol standpoint, is that egg whites are fat and cholesterol-free. You can eat them to your heart's content. You can enjoy egg whites anytime as part of a low-fat, cholesterol-reducing diet. And if your serum cholesterol is in the desirable range, you can throw in a highly nutritious egg yolk or two every so often, if you wish.

*You can enjoy egg whites anytime as part of a low-fat, cholesterol-reducing diet.*

## Putting It All Together

To achieve your healthy eating and weight goals once and for all:

1. about 55% of your total daily calories should come from carbohydrate, which is your burning fuel or gasoline

2. consume a moderate amount of protein food, about six ounces cooked per day, lean and well-trimmed, for building blocks

3. reduce your fat intake to no more than 30% of calories or less

## Carbo Caveat

Starchy foods like bread, pasta and potatoes used to be considered "fattening". They were probably the first foods people would eliminate when they were trying to reduce their weight. When the national food guides were revised emphasizing grains, vegetables and fruits, people started to become more comfortable with including starchy foods in their diets. Before long, the bagel became king. Pasta ruled supreme.

Lately, however, many have started to question this way of eating. The pendulum is swinging, once again, away from eating starchy foods. It seems that North Americans are not achieving their weight goals with their low-fat, high carbohydrate diets. Why is this happening?

The reason, in my opinion, is similar to the too much fat-free food scenario I talked about earlier. In my practice I've seen many clients who have unknowingly been overeating in the belief that starchy foods like pasta and bagels are healthy, naturally low in fat, and therefore low in calories. These foods are low in fat, but they can pack a real calorie-laden punch, especially when consumed in typical North American serving-size portions.

A large bagel or a restaurant helping of pasta, can easily add up to three or four starch servings or more. This may be fine for a growing, active teen with high energy needs. For a fairly sedentary woman or man trying to achieve a healthy weight, it can be too much.

I recently reviewed the diet history of a female client. She was eating a three-ounce bagel (equal to three starch servings) with light cream cheese and coffee for breakfast; another bagel (three starch servings) with tuna and salad for lunch; two cups of pasta (four starch servings) with chicken and tomato sauce for supper; and she munched on three cups of popcorn (one starch serving) as a snack in the evening. This added up to a whopping eleven servings of starch in one day. It could be even more if she got into the baked chips, rice cakes and low-fat cookies. She couldn't understand why her weight wouldn't budge, even though she was following a low-fat diet.

When we replaced her morning bagel with a serving of bran flakes, skim milk and a fruit, her lunch-time bagel with two slices of whole wheat bread, cut her pasta down to one cup, exchanged her popcorn for a fat-free yogurt and substituted more vegetables and fruit for some of the starch, she started seeing results. She now consumes about five to six starch servings per day, is eating a more balanced and satisfying menu, and is delighted with her progress.

I'll give you another example. A male client came to see me with the goal of reducing his weight. He was working out daily. He was consuming a high carbohydrate, low-fat diet to fuel his active lifestyle. He ate plenty of starchy foods like bagels, cereal, pasta and muffins. He couldn't understand why he too was gaining weight.

After reviewing his diet, I suspected that he was also overeating on starchy foods, at times at the expense of lean protein. A simple adjustment of lowering his starchy food intake, including at least six ounces of lean protein daily, increasing his vegetable intake, introducing fruit and yogurt as an evening snack while continuing to keep his fat intake low, helped him achieve his healthy weight goal. And the workouts continued to be better than ever.

A high carbohydrate diet means that a higher percentage of daily calories should come from carbohydrate, about 55%. It doesn't mean that starchy carbohydrate food intake should be sky high.

To reach your healthy eating and weight goals, consume less starchy foods if you've been overeating these foods. Substitute vegetables and fruits for some of the starch. They tend to be lower in calories, are nutritious and filling too. Choose more satisfying whole grains over white flour for their higher fiber content. And be sure to include a source of lean protein at your meals, which will help you stay fuller longer. Finally, be careful not to "out-eat" your workout, especially on starchy foods just because you're exercising regularly.

*To reach your healthy eating and weight goals, consume less starchy foods if you've been overeating these foods.*

## Water Works

You're probably surprised that I haven't yet mentioned the dreaded eight cups of water or more that you should be drinking every day. The time has come. You do need to drink water and I'll tell you why.

Our bodies are approximately 60% water, muscle tissue is about 70% water. Water is needed for most functions that take place in the body. You can survive several weeks without food, but far less without water. You need to replace the water that you're constantly losing in your perspiration, when you breathe and when you eliminate waste from the body. You need to drink about eight cups per day to keep you well hydrated and feeling refreshed.

Water is extremely helpful when you're trying to achieve your healthy eating and weight goals too. Aside from all its other virtues, water is filling and has zero calories and fat. If you haven't been drinking much water lately, start with a few cups or more and gradually build up to eight. Otherwise you may feel water-logged.

*Aside from all its other virtues, water is filling and has zero calories and fat.*

You can also get your water in the form of vegetables and fruits which are anywhere from 75-95% water, soups, herbal tea, hot water with lemon, decaf coffee, juices and diet soft drinks. Although caffeine acts as a diuretic by drawing water out of the body, some of the water in a caffeine-containing beverage is retained in the body. This is not the case with alcohol.

Get into the habit of drinking water. Keep a pitcher in the refrigerator so you'll choose water instead of a soft drink. Go for a water-break at work instead of the usual coffee-break. You'll be less tempted to have a donut or a Danish pastry. They don't go quite as well with water.

Sip water at your desk while you're working. It will lubricate your throat, especially if you do a lot of talking on the phone. Keep a water bottle with you whenever you're physically active, so you'll remember to drink before, during and after your workout. And be sure to include a soup or salad with your lunch and dinner. That's a really easy way to get extra fluid. You can do the quiz in Part 3 to help get you into the water habit.

*Keep a water bottle with you whenever you're physically active, so you'll remember to drink before, during and after your workout.*

# The 10 Most Fattening Foods
## And What You Can Eat Instead to Achieve Your Healthy Eating and Weight Goals

1.  **Coconut Oil (14 g fat/tbsp, 120 calories, 100% calories from fat)**

    Like all oils, coconut oil derives almost 100% of its calories from fat. But unlike most oils that are healthy when consumed in small amounts, coconut oil is solid at room temperature, is 92% saturated and can contribute to high cholesterol.

    Coconut oil is found in some processed foods, so be sure to read labels. Some movie theater popcorn may still be popped in coconut oil. This is a good reason to have a fruit or yogurt instead, before or after the show.

2.  **Butter (12 g fat/tbsp, 108 calories, 100% calories from fat)**

    Butter is another saturated fat. The fat from butter can easily be gobbled up by hungry fat cells and can potentially raise cholesterol levels. Top your baked potato with low-fat yogurt, fat-free sour cream, or a spicy salsa. Enjoy regular, Dijon or honey mustard on sandwiches and fruit spread on toast.

3.  **Margarine (11 g fat/tbsp, 100 calories, 100% calories from fat)**

    While lower in saturated fat than butter, margarine is also almost 100% fat. When choosing a margarine, go for one that is non-hydrogenated to avoid trans fat.

    To consume less fat, go for the same alternatives as for butter.

4.  **Mayonnaise (11 g fat/tbsp, 100 calories, 100% calories from fat)**

    Hold the mayo. A lean turkey, ham or roast beef sandwich is a better deli choice than tuna or chicken salad loaded with mayonnaise. For a rich and creamy taste and texture without the extra fat and calories, prepare tuna in the food processor with a dab of ultra-light mayo or fat-free yogurt.

5. **Macadamia Nuts (21g fat/oz, 199 calories, 95% calories from fat)**

Most nuts and seeds are high in fat, but macadamia nuts take the heavy-weight title. And for those of you who love peanut butter (75% calories from fat), peanut butter is generally a healthy choice, especially for an active child who needs the extra fat and calories for growth and development. For an adult trying to achieve a healthy weight, use sparingly as a fat choice or choose instead fruit spread or apple butter (0% fat) on toast or English muffins.

6. **Blue Cheese Salad Dressing (8 g fat/tbsp, 76 calories, 95% calories from fat)**

Most prepared salad dressings are high in fat and blue cheese is no exception. Instead, go for a squeeze of lemon and plenty of fresh-ground pepper, a flavored or seasoned vinegar, a low-fat or fat-free dressing, or ask for dressing on the side so you can choose how much you use.

7. **Cream Cheese (10 g fat/oz, 100 calories, 90% calories from fat)**

Make your own yogurt cheese by placing a strainer lined with a coffee filter over a bowl. Add fat-free yogurt. Place in refrigerator overnight and in the morning you'll have a light spread to enjoy on your toast. Or whip 1% cottage cheese in the food processor for a creamy low-fat cheese spread.

8. **Avocado, California (9.7 g fat/2 oz, 99 calories, 88% calories from fat)**

The avocado is one of the few vegetables that is high in fat. The olive is another. For a mouth-watering veggie sandwich, go light on the avocado and heavy on the layers of grated carrot, shredded lettuce, tomato slices, cucumber rings, sliced beets, purple onions and plenty of sprouts, piled high on a whole grain roll, slathered with spicy mustard. What a mouthful!

9. **Chicken Skin, roasted (12 g fat/oz, 129 calories, 84% calories from fat)**

Most of the fat in chicken is found in and just under the skin. Skinless chicken is a lower fat choice. Just pull off the skin or buy skinless chicken breasts at the supermarket.

When eating on the go, choose a grilled chicken sandwich on a bun (skip the mayo), or a roasted quarter-chicken without the skin or wing. Hold the fries. They can pack on 14 grams of fat or more per serving. Instead, have a steaming baked potato or crisp salad with low-fat dressing.

10. **Pepperoni (11g fat/oz, 126 calories, 79% calories from fat)**

Pepperoni, sausage and salami can boost the fat content of your favorite pizza through the roof. Choose low-fat toppings like mushrooms, green and red pepper rings, sliced tomatoes, onions or pineapple. When you make your own pizza at home, use the same healthy toppings and a sprinkle of part-skim Mozzarella cheese.

Some high fat runners-up include ice cream, fried foods, fatty cuts of meat, most cheeses, creamy sauces and rich desserts.

# CHAPTER 3

# The Lighter Weigh

WHEN IT COMES TO ACHIEVING a healthy weight, it can be pretty discouraging to think about reducing your weight by twenty, thirty, forty, fifty pounds or more. Sometimes, just thinking about these numbers, numbers that seem so big, can keep you from even trying.

But the good news is that even a modest weight reduction, say ten to fifteen pounds, can help lower cholesterol levels, improve blood sugar control in type 2 diabetics, reduce blood pressure if high, and show you that you really can do it.

So right now, instead of focusing on what your ultimate healthy weight goal should be, make a commitment to eat in a healthy way, to choose lower fat foods and to enjoy some new recipes. Dream big by thinking small: small changes, small attainable goals, fitting into some of your smaller clothes.

As you work toward achieving your healthy weight, aim to reduce your weight by about 1-2 pounds (0.5-1.0 kg) per week. Set a five to ten pound mini-goal for yourself. Give yourself that well-deserved pat on the back with a non-food reward when you achieve your goal.

One day, a client came to my office sporting her reward to herself. It was a trendy pair of boots that made her feel

*Dream big by thinking small: small changes, small attainable goals, fitting into some of your smaller clothes.*

absolutely fantastic. Plan a non-food reward for yourself too. It can be anything that makes you feel great, a token to yourself that says "I'm proud of Me".

When I was moving toward my healthy weight goal, my non-food reward was something new to wear. First I would study fashion magazines. Then I'd go shopping. Being able to fit into and look great in a new outfit, well that was a reward in itself.

What a change from those heart-wrenching days in my teens when shopping for clothes usually left me in tears. I'd either end up with nothing to buy or else would choose something, not because I liked it, but because it fit. Fortunately, I've been able to turn those painful memories into a happier today. And now, by maintaining my healthy weight for all these years, I've assembled a lovely wardrobe in one size that I love to wear each day. And so will you.

## Your Healthy Weight

When you're ready, follow the steps I take with my clients to see if you have a healthy weight, or to determine what your healthy weight goal should be.

When a new client comes to see me, I take a weight history which includes his/her lowest and highest adult weights. I need to know the client's current weight, so I ask my client to step up on the scale. This is, without question, the worst part of the visit.

Everyone, including me hates to be weighed. Years ago when I was seeing my dietitian, until she weighed me, I couldn't concentrate on a word she was saying. My heart would pound like a drum in my chest because I knew that any minute I would have to step on the scale. So now in my own practice, I get the weighing over with early. And I'm prepared for the usual reasons why the weight's not right (always too high). Check these out. Recognize any?

1. I forgot to take off my watch.
2. I just ate.
3. I didn't have time to go to the bathroom.
4. My scale at home is digital (therefore more accurate).
5. I'm wearing heavy underwear.
6. I'm bloated.
7. I ate Chinese/Japanese food last night.
8. The floor is tilted.
9. I just finished a triple latté.
10. It's before, during or after the time of the month. ( Also said by a male client whose wife eats more when she's premenstrual. She doesn't like to eat alone.)

Do these sound familiar? They certainly do to me. Not because I hear them every day, but because I've said them too, just like everybody else.

So why do I even bother to weigh my clients? I really wish I didn't have to. But the truth is, monitoring weight change does provide one measure of progress.

But it's only one. There are many other factors that are more important than the numbers on the scale. Enjoying balanced meals, making a new recipe, eating in response to body cues like hunger instead of emotions, making healthier food choices and discovering non-food rewards are the changes that really count.

*There are many other factors that are more important than the numbers on the scale.*

After I weigh my client, I calculate the Body Mass Index (BMI) to determine if my client has a healthy weight. If it is above a healthy weight, we talk about what lower weight has been maintained in the past. I ask this because I want my client to aim for a weight that is realistic, not some very low weight that may have been achieved on a fad diet but didn't last.

By using these numbers, along with other health, dietary and family history information, a healthy weight goal can be determined. This can take place in the first visit, but more often the weight goal is discussed when the client is ready and the time is right.

Before you can determine what your healthy weight goal should be, let's first talk about what it isn't. A healthy weight is not the lowest weight that you once starved yourself down to on a crash diet, or when you were chain smoking instead of eating, or that time you had a bad case of the flu.

Just like Oprah, who couldn't fit into those size ten jeans after she started eating real food instead of her liquid fasting diet, your all-time lowest weight may not be the most realistic weight for you either. When Oprah ultimately "made the connection" between a healthy lifestyle and a healthy weight, she was able to achieve and maintain her goals. And so will you.

A healthy weight is the one that is realistic for you. The following are six factors you need to consider:

## 1. Body Mass Index (BMI)

*You can calculate your BMI by dividing your weight in kilograms by your height in meters squared.*

The body mass index is a tool used for determining a healthy weight in adults. It assesses overall weight and health risk. You can calculate your BMI by dividing your weight in kilograms by your height in meters squared. This will tell you if your weight falls within the range that is considered healthy.

If your calculated BMI falls between 20 and 25, you generally have a healthy weight. Below 20 is considered underweight, between 25 and 27 indicates caution, and above 27 indicates an increased risk for health problems like heart disease, type 2 diabetes and some cancers.

There's quite a broad range of weights that is considered "healthy" for a given height. If your BMI is above 27, an initial goal should be to get within the healthy weight range. You can then use further information to fine-tune your ultimate weight goal.

## 2. Personal Weight History

Suppose you've calculated your BMI, and you find that it is 25. This is considered in the healthy weight range. But you know that you've recently gained 15 pounds. By reducing the weight you'll still be in the healthy range, but it will be a better weight for you because it is one at which you feel and look better, and you've been able to maintain this weight in the past.

You can use your personal weight history to determine what weight is not realistic for you, too. As a client put it, she ignores "ideal" weight charts, especially those in beauty magazines. Since she hasn't been a size 12 since she was twelve years old, she's not about to frustrate herself now by aiming for a size or weight that's not right for her. Trying to achieve an unrealistic weight goal will only make you feel unhappy and dissatisfied with yourself. Remember, you're an individual and what's theoretically "ideal" for someone else, may not be realistic for you.

*Trying to achieve an unrealistic weight goal it will only make you feel unhappy and dissatisfied with yourself.*

## 3. Family History

We know that body weight, like most physical characteristics is strongly influenced by genes. Identical twins, separated at birth and raised in different environments, tend to achieve and maintain very similar weights.

So take a look at your parents, grandparents, siblings, aunts and uncles. It will give you a good idea of what the weight

*Instead of eyeing that skinny pair of jeans at the mall, take a look at the genes that really matter.*

trends in your family are. Instead of eyeing that skinny pair of jeans at the mall, take a look at the genes that really matter.

That's not to say that you should adopt a fatalistic attitude and accept being overweight if you don't want to be, because it's a family trend. You can, and should, strive to be as healthy as you can be.

But take into account where you came from and the genetic forces you may need to overcome to achieve your goals. This will allow you to be realistic and avoid being disappointed with what you can or cannot accomplish.

## 4. Medical History

Certain medical conditions like high blood pressure, type 2 diabetes and high cholesterol can be improved with weight reduction. If you suffer from any of these conditions, even a modest drop of ten to fifteen pounds can help. Set a healthy weight goal with the help of your doctor. Consult a dietitian who can design a personal menu plan to help you reach your goals with appropriate food choices and lifestyle guidance.

## 5. Body fat Distribution

Are you an "apple" or a "pear"? Research suggests that those who store fat on their mid-sections, the people we call apples, may be at greater risk for health problems like heart disease, high cholesterol and triglycerides, type 2 diabetes and some cancers, than those whose body fat is stored on the hips and thighs. Those are the pears.

To determine if you're an apple or a pear, calculate your waist to hip ratio (WHR) by dividing your waist by your hip measurement. For women, a desirable ratio is no greater than 0.8, for men it is 1.0.

After you calculate your WHR, you can use this information to help determine what your healthy weight goal should be. If your WHR is higher than the desirable level, a plan to achieve the desired ratio is probably a good idea. If your body fat is stored mainly on the hips, although you may not be happy with your silhouette, it may not be as critical to your health to reduce your weight further.

## 6. How You Feel

The last factor you need to consider is how you feel. You probably thought I was going to say how you look, because this is one of the most common reasons people give for wanting to reduce their weight—to look better. But your health, energy level and feeling of well-being are what really count.

Being overweight can make you feel tired and sluggish. Even getting into and out of a car can be a major chore. With a healthy weight, everyday activities can be much easier to handle. Be sure to consider not only how you look but how you feel when deciding a weight goal that's right for you.

*But your health, energy level and feeling of well-being are what really count.*

# Keep the Following Tips In Mind When You Think About Your Healthy Weight Goal.

1. Focus on "achieving your healthy weight goal," not on "losing weight".

2. A healthy weight goal is one that you can achieve and maintain.

3. Aim for a weight reduction of about 1-2 pounds (0.5–1.0 kg) per week.

4. To get started, set a five to ten pound mini-goal.

5. Reward yourself when you achieve your mini-goal.

6. Determine your ultimate goal weight when you're ready.

7. Consider six factors in setting your goal.

8. Many lifestyle-related health problems can be improved with even a modest reduction in weight.

9. Body weight is influenced by genes.

10. A realistic healthy weight goal is more important than an "ideal" weight. Ask yourself, is this weight ideal for me?

## The Lighter Weigh

You'll need to follow these steps to determine your healthy weight goal:

1. calculate your BMI to determine if your weight is in the healthy range

2. record your lowest adult weight and how long you maintained this weight

3. figure your WHR to determine if you are an apple or a pear

4. review your family tree for possible weight trends

5. determine if you have any medical conditions that might be improved with a reduction in weight

6. assess your weight as it affects your feeling of well-being

When you're ready, use The Lighter Weigh tool in Part 3 to help you establish your healthy weight goal.

# CHAPTER 4

# Snack Attack Strategy

A "SNACK" CAN BE DEFINED as a small quantity of food, a light meal or refreshment taken between regular meals. Snacks, for example, are especially important for young children. Their small tummies can't hold much food, so snacks provide them with the between meal nourishment that they need. For adults, a snack hits the spot when a meal is delayed, when blood sugar starts to dip and energy starts to decline.

In North America however, "snacking" has become a pastime in itself, regardless of the need for food. There's even a snack food industry that churns out every conceivable form of munchie—chip, pretzel, cracker, cookie and candy. Does this sound like nourishment to you? I hope not.

Snacking in our culture is a form of entertainment. It's marketed as "fun". It's something to do when you're bored, anxious or frustrated, or when you're watching television or a movie, reading or surfing the net.

Snacking is often just something to do with your hands or your mouth. But, to your body, the fat and calories coming from this pasttime have only one place to go. Can you guess where? It brings to mind the saying "one minute on the lips, soon to be on the hips".

> *Snacking in our culture is a form of entertainment. It's marketed as "fun".*

A client called me one day to asked me if it was okay for her to have popcorn at the movies. I asked her if she thought she was going to be hungry while she watched the show. She said probably not. My answer therefore was a simple "No".

The reason I say "no" to eating popcorn at the movies, is that, like munching chips while watching TV or nibbling candy while reading, it's a good habit to break.

Even though most movie theater popcorn is being popped with a healthier fat, canola oil, instead of that most saturated fat, coconut oil, and even though air-popped popcorn can be relatively low in fat and calories, my answer is still "no".

Now before you dismiss me as the wicked witch of the popcorn counter, let me explain. The popcorn itself isn't necessarily "bad" or "good". Remember, we talked about that earlier. There are no good or bad foods. It's the eating behavior that matters.

Suppose every time you go to a movie you absolutely must have a bag of popcorn. With the size of the mega-bags of popcorn sold at the multi-plexes these days, that can add up to hundreds of extra calories that your body probably doesn't need.

Like most people, you become conditioned to associate going to the movies with eating popcorn. Before you know it, you start to salivate for popcorn as soon as you enter a movie theater. Movie means popcorn. Who cares if the movie is bad, at least I got the popcorn.

Next time you're at the movies, look around to see how many people have fallen into this habit. The more engrossed they become in the movie, the less aware they are of how much popcorn they're actually consuming. The more heated the action gets on the screen or the more tense the plotline, the more popcorn gets eaten.

At home, suppose you always snack on chips, pretzels or nuts when you watch TV. Watching TV won't seem right

*Before you know it, you start to salivate for popcorn as soon as you enter a movie theater.*

unless you have a bowl of chips or bag of something to munch on. I have many a client who wrestle with this problem all the time. If you're in the habit of eating candy while you're reading, you'd better have a king-size supply of candy handy if you're reading a book you can't put down.

Be on the alert. Going to the movies, watching TV and reading a book can be fattening, if you combine these pastimes with nibbling, munching and snacking.

When you eat, just eat. Don't eat and watch movies or TV. Don't dine and and drive. Instead put food purchases in the trunk. Don't munch and chat on the phone. It's rude to talk with your mouth full anyway. Don't nibble and prepare dinner. Chew a piece of sugarless gum instead. Don't graze and work on the computer. Eat when you're hungry and do only that.

Set a welcoming place for yourself in your kitchen or in your dining room. Enjoy your food. If you're eating alone, put on some background music. Relax and savor the delicious food you've prepared for yourself. After you're finished, go ahead and watch your movie, read your book or talk on the phone.

And please, always sit down to eat. Even though we'd love to believe that the calories consumed while we're standing don't count, they sure do. That includes nibbling while cooking or clearing the table, munching straight from the refrigerator, cupboard or freezer, and grazing over the counter or sink. (If you're wondering how I know all this, it's because I've done it all too.)

Now you're probably wondering, "What if I really want a snack while I'm watching TV or reading my book?" Then follow these steps my clients and I take to successfully handle a snack attack.

*Even though we'd love to believe that the calories consumed while we're standing don't count, they sure do.*

# Snack Attack Strategy

1. Ask yourself "Am I hungry?"

2. If the answer is "yes", prepare a satisfying snack from the snack list.

3. Place the food on a plate and enjoy eating your snack, sitting at a table.

4. Do not take your snack to the den, to your desk or to the bedroom. Establish non-eating zones. By that I mean any room other than the kitchen or dining room. Just think, no more crumbs to vacuum up.

5. Never eat your snack while you're watching television, doing work or reading a book. If you do, you'll want to keep eating as long as you're doing that activity. It's easy to slip into mindless eating when you're doing other things.

6. When you're finished your snack, put your plate away and leave the kitchen.

7. If you weren't hungry to begin with, try to determine if you're bored, anxious, frustrated or you're just used to snacking while watching television, reading or working.

8. Once you realize that the desire to snack is probably just a habit, distract yourself by going to a non-eating zone such as the bedroom, living room, or study. This really works. You'll see how quickly the desire to eat will leave you as soon as you go to a room where you don't usually eat.

9. Plan non-snacking activities such as calling a friend, going for a walk, giving yourself a facial or manicure, pruning your plants, clipping your nails, balancing your chequebook, playing with the dog, or washing the car for those non-hungry snack urges.

10. Pat yourself on the back for successfully handling your snack attack. It will be easier the next time.

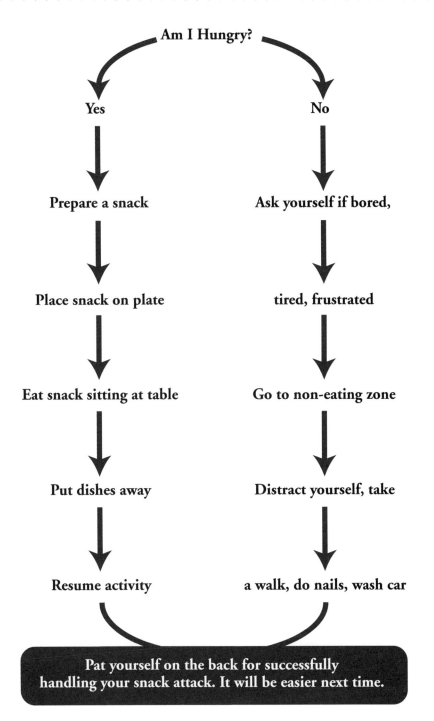

**Am I Hungry?**

| Yes | No |
|-----|-----|
| Prepare a snack | Ask yourself if bored, |
| Place snack on plate | tired, frustrated |
| Eat snack sitting at table | Go to non-eating zone |
| Put dishes away | Distract yourself, take |
| Resume activity | a walk, do nails, wash car |

Pat yourself on the back for successfully handling your snack attack. It will be easier next time.

## 10 Light Snacks for When You're Truly Hungry

1. ½ cup fruit salad, 2 tbsp fat-free yogurt, 1 tbsp. wheat germ
2. 1 cup spicy clamato juice, 2 celery stalks, 2 melba rounds
3. ½ cup cereal, ½ cup skim milk, ½ cup sliced strawberries
4. 2 egg whites on toast, sliced tomato
5. 1 cup lite hot chocolate, 2 arrowroot biscuits
6. 1 cup veggies with ¼ cup yogurt dip
7. 1 oz baked chips with ¼ cup salsa
8. 1 low-fat muffin, 1 cup herbal tea
9. 1 cup gazpacho or cauliflower soup, 2 soda crackers
10. 1 slice whole grain toast, 2 tbsp yogurt cheese, 1tsp fruit spread

## Beware of "Multiples"

Be careful when you eat anything that is sold in a bag or a box like cookies or crackers, or is served in a bowl like potato chips, popcorn, nuts or pretzels. I call these "multiples" because we can't eat just one or two. We devour them in multiples of two or more. I've composed a rhyme that goes with multiples:

"Two and four and six and eight,
How will I achieve a healthy weight?"

We eat multiples until all the broken ones are gone, the bag is empty, the bowl is clean and the box is finished. The ads are right. We can't eat just one.

And I've figured out why. Once the multiple-to-mouth motion starts, it's hard to stop, especially when we're stressed, tired or bored. Eating multiples seems to induce a hypnotic trance in which we continue to munch in a robot-like way.

To avoid falling into this state, you're better off having a satisfying mini-meal as a snack. However, if you are one of the few that can consume a multiple in a pre-measured or pre-counted portion using the snack attack strategy, then go ahead. But if you're tempted to go for more, stick to your real food snacks next time.

I understand this very well because I too went through many a bag and box of multiples in my chronic dieting days. I still find it hard to avoid the multiple trance whenever I'm tempted to eat pretzels, cookies or baked chips. In most cases, I've found it's better not to start.

> *Eating multiples seems to induce a hypnotic trance in which we continue to munch in a robot-like way.*

CHAPTER 5

# *Norman the "Nutritionist"*

*I*'D LIKE TO INTRODUCE you to Norman the "Nutritionist". He's not really a nutritionist. He's my husband. So you're probably wondering what he's doing in this book. He actually didn't want me to write about him, but I couldn't resist.

Along with helping me get started on a healthier lifestyle and encouraging me daily to fulfill my dreams, Norman is one of those rare and fortunate people who instinctively knows how to eat in a healthy way. And he usually does. I can assure you he's really quite a lovable guy, even though he makes healthy eating look easy while the rest of us have to work so hard at it.

I started calling Norman a nutritionist after I went back to university to study food and nutrition. Much to his supreme satisfaction, I learned that many of his natural eating and lifestyle habits were the very ones that most of us were trying so hard to achieve. You probably know a few natural "nutritionists" too. And you may also have some healthy habits that come naturally to you too.

Let's take a look at what Norman does and see how his instincts add up to a healthy lifestyle.

> *I started calling Norman a nutritionist after I went back to university to study food and nutrition.*

## Norman the "Nutritionist":

### • always eats breakfast

It's usually a balanced breakfast of whole grain cereal, skim milk and orange juice with lots of pulp. That way he starts the day off right and gets a head start on his intake of fiber, calcium and vitamin C.

On the weekend, he'll enjoy a brunch of bagels, herring, lox, light cream cheese and freshly squeezed orange juice. He picks up this feast on his way home from jogging at the park. He didn't need me to tell him that higher fat fish like salmon and herring contain heart healthy omega-3 fatty acids. He just eats what he likes.

### • eats when he's hungry, stops when he's full

How lucky can you get! Many years ago we were invited to join a group of friends who were going to an "all you can eat" buffet. I knew he'd probably be overwhelmed by all the food and come back from the buffet table with maybe a pickle or an olive on his plate. But to be sociable I accepted the invitation.

As our friends attacked the buffet, I soon lost sight of Norman. When I came back to the table, I still didn't see him. I was starting to get worried, so I asked one of his buddies to check out the washroom to see if he was there.

I found out later that sure enough, Norman got carried away eating and trying to keep up with the rest of the group. He started feeling unwell and headed to the washroom for relief. Unable to handle so much food so quickly, his body rebelled and made him stop.

Needless to say, we rarely go to "all you can eat" buffets any more. Norman usually knows his limit and he's wise to

*Unable to handle so much food so quickly, his body rebelled and made him stop.*

stick to it. Otherwise his body sends him a message he can't ignore.

### • usually has a bigger lunch, lighter supper

When we were first married, I couldn't understand why Norman wasn't terribly interested in the dinners that I was so eager to prepare for him. I admit that I wasn't the greatest cook in those days, but there had to be more to it than that. Or was there?

*I finally learned the truth after my Miami ribs fiasco.*

I finally learned the truth after my Miami ribs fiasco. Wanting to please, I tried making a dish suggested by the butcher. He guaranteed success. He told me to broil Miami short ribs, slathered with BBQ sauce, which I did in our tiny kitchen. Needless to say, my good intentions literally went up in smoke as our apartment filled with black clouds that came billowing from the oven. I was in tears. Norman said not to worry. He wasn't really hungry anyway.

And he wasn't just trying to spare my feelings. He truly wasn't hungry for dinner because he liked eating a larger meal at lunch. All he wanted for supper was a tunafish sandwich. With the way I cooked in those days, it was probably a safer choice, in more ways than one.

Most North Americans tend to skip breakfast, grab a fast bite for lunch and end up eating a huge meal at dinner and snack food all evening long. Norman, on the other hand, is usually hungriest and eats his biggest meal at lunch when his body needs the fuel for the rest of the day. He eats a lighter meal later on when his metabolism and activity level are slowing down.

### • can handle "multiples"

How many times have you opened a bag of potato chips, sat down to watch a TV show and before you knew it, all the chips were gone? That's because to most of us, chips are "multiples". We eat them until there are none left.

Not Norman the Nutritionist. Unlike the rest of us, when he gets a craving for chips, he can eat a handful, roll up the bag and put them away. He's been warned. Around our house, if he buys chips and expects to see them again anytime in the near future, he'd better hide them in a safe place, away from the rest of us.

## • works out 3 times a week

I credit Norman with one of the biggest lifestyle changes that I've made. With his encouragement, I starting working out on a regular basis. This was certainly a big leap for me, tormented as I was by painful memories of having to jump over the dreaded boxhorse in gym class.

Norman jogs, lifts weights and often does some sit-ups with an ab-roller when he watches TV. When I started working out, he told me to stop jumping in aerobics class because it wasn't good for my joints. He encouraged me to do some training with weights. He even offered to be my personal trainer. He believed that I could get an excellent cardiovascular workout with low-impact aerobics and that weight training would strengthen my muscles and tone my body. Good advice.

*This was certainly a big leap for me, tormented as I was by painful memories of having to jump over the dreaded boxhorse in gym class.*

## • takes every opportunity to watch a funny show, listen to a comedy tape, tell a joke and laugh out loud

Laughter is the best medicine, something that Norman has always known. When he visits someone who is sick, what does he bring? Not the usual flowers, plant or candy. He shows up with a comedy tape, a book of jokes or a funny movie to make his friend really feel better. And you know, it usually works.

A recent study showed that only thirty minutes a day of "mirthful laughter" resulted in a decline in the recurrence of heart attacks in patients who had already suffered one heart attack. Stress can depress the immune system. Laughter can reduce stress hormones in the body by as much as 50%.

When I told Norman about the study, he said "of course", and continued watching one of his favorite TV shows, a rerun of the Jack Benny program.

So take a tip from Norman. If you're feeling stressed, anxious or bored, go for a good laugh instead of something to eat.

*If you're feeling stressed, anxious or bored, go for a good laugh instead of something to eat.*

### • changes out of his business suit at the end of the day, puts on a shirt, jeans and a belt to relax in

Most people relax in a pair of sweat-pants and a loose fitting shirt. Not Norman. He can be seen relaxing at home in his usual ensemble—shirt, jeans and belt. What does this have to do with food and eating, you're wondering? Everything.

What sweat-pants have that jeans don't is an elasticized waistband that will expand to accommodate almost any quantity of food intake or weight gain. Save those loose fitting clothes for the gym. You don't want to put your waistline at risk. Wear something fitted and tucked in whenever you can instead of those expandable clothes that forgive and let us forget our healthy eating goals.

### • seldom eats popcorn at the movies anymore

We often go to a four o'clock movie on the weekend. We usually have a bite to eat after and play amateur movie critic as we review the show.

When Norman used to eat popcorn at the movies, he wasn't hungry for dinner afterwards. This didn't make me very happy because I was usually starving and looking forward to going out to eat. We couldn't figure out why he was getting so full on the popcorn. Wasn't popcorn supposed to be a healthy, low-fat and low calorie snack food?

We soon found out that most movie theater popcorn was popped in that most saturated fat, coconut oil, and plenty of it. No wonder Norman couldn't eat after the show. He was full from the fat and calories in the popcorn.

These days, movie theater popcorn is mostly popped in healthier canola oil. But you'll still get lots of fat and calories, especially if you go for those mega-tubs that can hold several cups or more.

Thankfully, Norman seldom eats popcorn at the movies anymore. And I get to enjoy a nice dinner after the show.

## • usually has fruit for dessert

At the end of a meal, Norman will often go for an apple, grapefruit or an orange for dessert. Because he seems to make so many healthy food choices naturally, I sometimes wonder what his body is craving.

Is it the soluble fiber that helps lower cholesterol? Maybe it's the anti-oxidant power of the vitamin C. Knowing him as I do, he probably just likes the taste. Whatever it is, Norman and I both agree that fruit is nature's dessert. It makes a great ending to a healthy meal.

> *Norman and I both agree that fruit is nature's dessert. It makes a great ending to a healthy meal.*

## • doesn't feel guilty when he eats ice cream or chocolate

Lest you wonder by now if Norman is human (and how much more of this you can take), let me assure you that just like the rest of us, he loves ice cream and chocolate.

*Remember, there are no good or bad foods. It's all about choice, balance and moderation.*

And every so often, he satisfies his sweet tooth and doesn't feel one bit guilty.

Instead, without thinking about it, he'll naturally balance the extra fat and calories with lighter choices at his next meal. He listens to his body and that's what I want you to do. Remember, there are no good or bad foods. It's all about choice, balance and moderation.

## So What Can We Learn From Norman the "Nutritionist"?

1. Always eat breakfast.

2. Eat when you're hungry, stop when you're full.

3. Eat more of your food earlier in the day when your body needs it.

4. Avoid multiples if you can't eat just a few.

5. Combine regular physical activity with healthy eating.

6. Laugh every day as often as you can.

7. Expandable waistbands are hazardous to your waistline.

8. Beware of hidden fat and calories in movie theater popcorn.

9. Fruit is nature's dessert.

10. If you eat a higher fat food, don't feel guilty, just balance it with a lighter choice.

# CHAPTER 6

# The Light Stuff

J ust like the astronauts you're going to need the right stuff...the light stuff, to help you on your mission to achieve your healthy eating goals. And where will you find the light stuff? Just blast off to the supermarket.

Supermarkets really do live up to their names. They're super in every sense of the word—size, food choices and convenience. And while they may seem like a galaxy of temptation to someone trying to reduce fat and calories, remember, they also offer a universe of healthy choices too. Fresh vegetables and fruits, cereals, grains and baked goods, skim dairy products, leaner meats, poultry and fish and countless lower fat and fat-free food products will help make your healthy eating goal a dream come true. What better place to get all-inspired and revved up about what you're doing?

But beware, supermarket shoppers. Never go food shopping on an empty stomach or without a shopping list. Cookies will cry out your name. Ice cream will sing its seductive song. Bags of potato chips will all but leap into your basket by themselves. So have a meal or snack before you go to make sure you stick to the light stuff. Remember, if you plan ahead, you won't leave yourself vulnerable to temptation.

*Never go food shopping on an empty stomach or without a shopping list.*

## Go for Vegetables and Fruit First

I like to shop at a supermarket that prides itself on its produce. This lets me know me what the store values most—fresh, wholesome, and healthy foods. A market that places more emphasis on real food rather than on countless aisles crammed with boxed and packaged products is the place for you and me.

Start your trip through the supermarket in the produce section. I guarantee you'll get excited about healthy eating when you see nature's dazzling array of wonderful colors, shapes and textures.

For your salads, choose some interesting greens, juicy tomatoes, firm cucumbers, shiny red, yellow and green sweet peppers, fresh green onions and crunchy radishes. Be daring. Get acquainted with a veggie you've never met before.

*Be daring. Get acquainted with a veggie you've never met before.*

For soups and your general cooking needs, include some Spanish onions, carrots, celery stalks, Italian parsley, potatoes, fragrant garlic and exotic ginger.

Richly-colored summer and winter squash, deep green broccoli, mushrooms, sugar-sweet snow peas and juicy bean sprouts add a boost of taste, texture and nutrition. Make a point to experiment with a new and different choice every week or two.

If you're shopping for one or two, pare down the quantities and some of the variety. Prepared salad greens and cut-up vegetables are available for those who don't have the time to wash and chop salads from scratch. You pay a little more for convenience, but you may actually save money by not having to throw away unused salad greens that end up languishing uneaten in the crisper.

Frozen vegetables are also a great alternative when you know that fresh produce won't be practical. Frozen peas, carrots and corn are fine, but try some of the newer medleys that offer variety with broccoli, cauliflower, zucchini and snow peas.

I've recently become a great tofu fan. The soy protein found in tofu contains a host of healthful phyto (plant) chemicals which may be protective against heart disease and cancer, and may even ease menopausal symptoms. If you haven't eaten tofu or soy products before, I bet you'll be as pleasantly surprised as I was at how versatile and tasty these foods really are. For starters, you can pick up a container of soft tofu which you can use in my tofu lasagna, some fat-free tofu cheese, soy "bologna" or "turkey" slices for sandwiches and a package of soy hot dogs or burgers to grill on the BBQ. Lite tofu is also available.

Stock up on fresh fruits in season. Apples and oranges are great portable fruits. Be sure to pick up a juicy cantaloupe or honeydew melon, succulent berries, golden pineapple and a fuzzy kiwi. You can cut up these luscious fruits, place them in a bowl and top with a splash of orange juice. Enjoy your fruit salad as an anytime snack or nature's own dessert.

Keep a bowl of fresh fruit on your kitchen counter as a reminder to go for a delicious fruit treat anytime. After supper be sure to bring out that wonderful fruit salad you made, so you'll have a satisfying ending to your evening meal. For variety, you can top your fruit salad with a dollop of fat-free yogurt.

*Keep a bowl of fresh fruit on your kitchen counter as an invitation to enjoy a delicious fruit treat anytime.*

## Dairy Delights

Choose skim or 1% milk, yogurt, cottage cheese and sour cream. I usually keep some shredded part-skim Mozzarella on hand for a low-fat pizza or veggie lasagna. When you buy hard cheese, choose 15% milkfat or less and ask for the cheese thinly sliced. Low-fat versions of feta and grated parmesan cheese are also handy for salad or pasta toppings. Low-fat soy drinks can be blended with fruit as a healthy smoothie or enjoyed with your favorite breakfast cereal. If the egg cooler is nearby, be sure to stock up on a carton or two of egg whites.

## Meat of the Matter

Let's review the Fab Four. It will help you make wise choices. Choose lean and well-trimmed meats, use a low-fat cooking method, keep portions to about 3 ounces (100 g) cooked weight, and enjoy a variety of meat, fish, poultry and alternatives.

Keeping this in mind, stock up on leaner cuts of meat, skinless, boneless chicken breasts, and some extra lean ground beef, veal or poultry for meatballs, pasta sauce or meatloaf. One pound (500 g) of ground will serve four to six. Try a new kind of fish. Ask the person working the counter to make a recommendation.

At the deli section, choose low-fat roasted turkey or chicken breast slices, lean ham or roast beef for sandwiches. Ask for the low sodium variety if available. "Roasted" is generally a healthier choice than "smoked".

## The Bread Basket

*When buying bagels, go for the smaller two-ounce size so your bagel will be equal to two bread servings.*

Choose sliced whole grain breads, rolls, bagels, pita or English muffins. One bread serving is generally equivalent to one ounce (30 g). When buying bagels, go for the smaller two-ounce size so your bagel will be equal to two bread servings. A large, twister bagel that weighs 6 ounces (and I've weighed them) is equal to 6 slices of bread.

## Awhile in the Aisles

Most of the fresh foods are generally found on the outer rim of the store. Up and down the aisles you'll find the packaged food products. This is where you'll need to be a label reader. And you won't be the only one with your reading glasses on.

Shoppers are becoming more savvy these days. Food stores are looking more and more like libraries these days with everyone studying the sides of cans and boxes. I want you to join them. Knowing how to read a food label will make a big difference when it comes to making healthy choices. There are three places to look for nutrition information.

## 1. Front of the package

Nutrition claims are usually found on the front of a food package as an enticement for the consumer to buy the food product. There are specific guidelines as to what these claims mean. For example, a product that says it is "cholesterol-free", must also be low in saturated fat. But don't start loading up your cart yet. After all, potato chips are cholesterol-free. Beware, the product may still be high in total and potentially artery-clogging trans fat, so you'll need to read further.

## 2. Ingredient list

Ingredients are listed in descending order from most to least plentiful. If some type of fat is listed as one or more of the first three ingredients, then there's a good chance the product is high in fat.

*If some type of fat is listed as one or more of the first three ingredients, then there's a good chance the product is high in fat.*

## 3. Nutrition information panel

At the present time, nutrition information labelling is voluntary in Canada. In the U.S., the nutrition facts must appear on a food label. Whenever the nutrition information is provided, check it out.

Let's calculate the percentage of calories coming from fat in this sample food, unsweetened peanut butter. The Nutrition Information label will look something like this:

## Nutrition Information
### per 14 g serving (1 tbsp)

| | |
|---|---|
| Energy | 96 calories |
| Protein | 4.0 g |
| Fat | 8.0 g |
| Carbohydrate | 2.0 g |
| Sugars | 0.4 g |
| Sodium | 1 mg |
| Potassium | 93 mg |

First, let's look at the amount of fat per serving. It's 8 grams. If we multiply the total fat, 8 grams by 9 calories per gram (each gram of fat provides 9 calories), you see that 72 calories in this serving comes from fat. When we divide the number of fat calories, 72, by the total number of calories per serving, which is 96, we find that a whopping 75% of the calories in this peanut butter comes from fat.

## Figuring the Fat

8 g of fat x 9 calories per gram = 72 calories from fat
72 calories divided by 96 total calories per serving = 0.75
0.75 x 100% = 75% of calories coming from fat

When clients ask me if they should have peanut butter on their breakfast toast, I point out how much fat they're getting. Peanut butter is a nutritious food for children who need the extra fat and calories for growth and development. But for an adult woman or man trying to reduce their weight, a lighter choice would be fruit spread on toast and a glass of skim milk or a fat-free yogurt for protein. A second option is to spread the peanut butter thinly, perhaps a 1-2 tsp serving size and count it as a fat choice.

You can use the "figuring the fat" formula to calculate the percentage of calories from fat. As I mentioned earlier, it is recommended that you consume no more than 30% of daily calories from fat. This formula can help you identify some of the more fattening foods, although not all foods can be expected to provide less than 30% calories from fat. You'll have a chance to practise your "figuring" in Part 3, Personal Journal.

## Healthy Fats

For cooking and food preparation, you'll need to buy some healthy fats. These include cooking spray, which comes in regular, butter and olive oil flavors, and olive oil for Mediterranean dishes. Canola, safflower, sunflower, soybean or corn oils are milder tasting options. If you use margarine, choose a non-hydrogenated type. Light varieties have some air or water whipped in. They can be used for cooking but are generally not recommended for baking.

*If you use margarine, choose a non-hydrogenated type.*

## Condiments, Spices and Herbs

Be sure to keep your refrigerator and pantry stocked with a good supply of flavored mustards and vinegars, salsa, ultra-light mayonnaise, fresh or dried herbs and spices. These contribute a lot of flavor, with little or no added fat and calories.

## Cereals

Nutrition information printed on breakfast cereals is based on a standard 30 gram (1 oz) serving size. This is good to know since all bowls of cereal aren't created equal.

For instance, a 30 gram serving of crispy rice cereal measures about 1 cup, and provides 110 calories and less than one gram of fat. A 30 gram serving of a granola-type cereal measures ¼ cup and provides 127 calories and 4 grams of fat.

At first glance this might not seem like much of a difference. But since most people eat at least 1 cup of cereal in their bowl, it means that a 1 cup bowl of granola cereal can pack a whopping 508 calories and 16 grams of fat.

*Don't assume that the information provided is for a "bowl" of cereal.*

This might be fine for a mountain climber hiking in the the Swiss Alps, but for a sedentary office worker, it's probably too much. So read cereal labels carefully. Aim for no more than 1 gram fat and less than 5 grams sugar per serving.

What about cereal bars? Are they a healthy choice? If it means that you'd be eating no breakfast at all or grabbing a donut and coffee instead, I'd certainly recommend the option of a cereal bar and a carton of skim milk. But when you have time to enjoy your breakfast at home, a cup of hot or cold cereal or a slice of whole grain toast, fresh fruit and skim milk or yogurt make for a balanced and satisfying start to your day.

## Crackers, Cookies, Snack Foods

Now we're getting into the realm of the "multiples". You read about multiples in the chapter called "Snack Attack Strategy". To review, multiples are foods that come in bags, boxes and packages. A good rule of thumb is to look for those that provide less than 1-2 grams of fat per serving. Keep a minimum of these foods in your cupboard.

Some acceptable choices include melba toast, (which I've started enjoying again after years of disliking them because of their past association with deprivation diets), arrowroot biscuits, graham wafers, Swedish flatbread, baked chips, pretzels, microwave light popcorn and rice cakes.

When it comes to these items, please commit these words to memory: NEVER EAT THESE FOODS FROM THE BAG OR BOX. Like the ad says, "Bet you can't eat just one." Before you know it, you'll end up eating two, four, six servings or more. Read the label to determine the serving size (which usually isn't very much), count out your portion and then put the bag or box away. Check out my Snack Attack Strategy for more tips.

*Read the label to determine the serving size (which usually isn't very much), count out your portion and then put the bag or box away.*

## Frozen Foods

You might want to pick up a bag of frozen mixed vegetables to keep in the freezer to toss into an egg white frittata, lasagna, stir-fry, pasta sauce or homemade soup. Zap your frozen veggies in the microwave and enjoy them on their own as a satisfying side dish. Frozen fish fillets and chicken breasts are also great to keep on hand for a quick supper.

I often recommend individual low-fat frozen yogurt or ice milk bars, especially the chocolate flavor, to help satisfy an ice cream or chocolate craving. Because they come individually wrapped, you can enjoy just one instead of having to resist a large container of frozen yogurt or ice milk calling to you from the freezer. If the frozen bars become multiples for you, you may have to avoid having them in the house for now.

## Canned Goods

Cans of crushed tomatoes, with or without added salt, water-packed tuna, fruit packed in its own juice, canned chickpeas, beans and lentils are terrific staples to keep on hand for light meals in a flash. Generally, other canned vegetables are less desirable because of their high sodium content.

## Soft Drinks, Beverages, Juices

You might want to stock up on sugar-free soft drinks, mineral or bottled water, herbal teas, decaf tea and coffee, and some fruit and vegetable juices to help meet your goal of drinking eight cups of fluid per day.

All beverages contribute to your daily fluid intake. Caffeine and alcohol act as diuretics that remove fluid from the body instead of replenishing it. Recent evidence, however, suggests that part of the fluid, perhaps as much as 50% in a caffeine-containing beverage is retained by the body and can contribute to your total daily fluid intake. This is not the case with alcohol.

## Light Stuff Shopping List

*Use the list whenever you go shopping to avoid impluse buying.*

To help you choose the light stuff the next time you go food shopping, use the handy Light Stuff Shopping List found in Part 3, Personal Journal. I've included items that you'll want to have on hand for the "Recipes for Success". Add your own needs to the list in the space that says "Other". Use the list whenever you go shopping to avoid impluse buying. And don't forget to have a healthy meal or snack before you hit the aisles.

# CHAPTER 7

# Enlightened Cooking

RATHER THAN TRYING to find all new healthy recipes that you and your family will enjoy, you can create lighter versions of your own favorites by following these simple tips.

When a recipe calls for browning vegetables such as onion, celery or carrot in oil, butter or margarine, cook on medium heat using a non-stick pan. Spray the pan with vegetable cooking spray and soften the vegetables in a little water or broth. For every tablespoon of oil you avoid, you'll be saving 14 grams of fat.

Bake, broil, steam, poach, microwave, BBQ or stir-fry food in a non-stick pan. If you don't own a good set of non-stick cookware, start with a non-stick frying pan and a medium-sized pot. Add to your collection as the need arises. One of my favorites is my 8-inch non-stick pan which turns out perfect egg white dishes. You'll also love having a non-stick grillpan for grilling foods indoors all year round.

Regular ground meat can be used to make lighter meat-based spaghetti sauce if you brown the meat first in your non-stick pot, pour off the fat, rinse the browned meat with warm water, and then continue with your recipe. You can wash away much of the fat with this method and forgo the expense of buying extra-lean ground meat. Do use extra-lean

*For every tablespoon of oil you avoid, you'll be saving 14 grams of fat.*

ground for meatloaf, meatballs or any dish where you can't drain or rinse off the fat.

Choose recipes that use meat, chicken or fish as an ingredient rather than as the main event. Plan meals around stir-fry dishes, stews, kebobs, wraps and fajitas instead of steaks and roasts. This is also an inexpensive way of extending the protein part of the meal and stretching your food dollar. It's good for your wallet and your waistline.

To cook vegetables, steam quickly or microwave in a little water to retain vitamins, minerals, color and crunch. For added flavor, add sliced fresh ginger, garlic or a little lite soy sauce to the cooking water. Turn out creamy smooth mashed potatoes by whipping in some of the cooking water instead of butter.

When baking muffins, use a minimum of oil, and substitute fruit juice, applesauce, prune purée, skim milk or yogurt for much of the fat. To retain moisture, freeze your low-fat muffins. With less fat, they will become stale more quickly. Take your muffins out of the freezer one at a time and zap in the microwave for a fresh-baked flavor and aroma.

You can make virtually fat-free soups, stews and gravies by refrigerating until the fat hardens on the surface, removing the hardened fat and then reheating before serving. If you're in a hurry, foods can be placed in the freezer for 20-30 minutes. This will make the fat congeal at the surface for easy removal.

Be creative with herbs and spices to cut back on the amount of salt you use. When using canned vegetables like chickpeas or kidney beans in a recipe, drain and rinse well with water. Add little, if any, salt to your recipe.

Serve lower fat, lighter fare the next time guests come for dinner. They'll appreciate your thoughtfulness, won't miss the extra fat and calories and you won't be left with high-fat food after the party's over.

## Pantry Staples

To be an enlightened cook, you'll need a supply of pantry staples so you can whip up something fast, healthy and delicious even when you're in a hurry. I love to cook but I don't have a lot of time to spend in the kitchen. I'm happy to take a few healthy shortcuts whenever I can. Now, I'm happy to share them with you.

The following are some terrific staples that you'll need to prepare the "Recipes for Success" and to lighten up your own cooking. I've mentioned several of these foods before, but it doesn't hurt to review.

## Dried herbs and spices

It's great to use fresh whenever you can. Why not plant a small herb garden in the spring or start a few pots on the windowsill? Or if you're really pressed for time, do what I do. Keep a good supply of dried herbs handy. My favorites include dried parsley, basil, oregano, tarragon, thyme, rosemary and cilantro. Many of my recipes call for the dried variety, but by all means, use fresh if you have them. Generally 1 tsp of dried herbs is equivalent to 2 tbsp of fresh.

*My favorites include dried parsley, basil, oregano, tarragon, thyme, rosemary and cilantro.*

Seasonings and seasoning blends are very helpful too. Garlic powder, cayenne, chili powder, and cumin, and Italian, Tex-Mex and BBQ seasonings are all handy. Many blends contain salt. Check the label and use little if any added salt if you use these blends.

## Frozen mixed vegetables, bagged salad mixes

As with herbs and seasonings, use fresh whenever possible. But when you don't have time to shop, wash and chop, frozen vegetables are a convenient alternative. They come in wonderful varieties like California, Italian and Oriental. I especially like California vegetables puréed in a velvety vegetable soup, I use the Italian in pasta with chicken, and the Oriental tastes great tossed into a tofu stir-fry.

Many of my clients who live alone wouldn't otherwise be eating a variety of vegetables if they didn't keep a good supply of the frozen on hand. So take a tip from them. This goes for the bagged salad mixes too. You pay a little more for the convenience, but it's worth it.

## Canned beans, peas and lentils

As a time-saver, I use canned beans, peas and lentils most often in recipes. Drained and rinsed canned chickpeas sprinkled with freshly ground black pepper are terrific as a quick and easy appetizer. Or you can make a healthy hummus by blending chickpeas in the food processor with a little ultra-light mayonnaise, lemon juice, a bit of tahini and seasonings. Along with other varieties of beans, they're a great source of protein when added to salads and soups.

With a can of black beans and a can of corn niblets, both drained and rinsed, you can impress your friends with a black bean and corn salad with fresh cilantro and diced red bell pepper. Your salad will look like it belongs on the cover of a gourmet magazine and you'll look like a gastronomic genius.

To cut down on salt, always drain and rinse canned beans. Use little, if any, salt in your recipe.

## Dried pasta, rice, barley, kasha, couscous

Pastas and grains are always ready and waiting to go into a pot of boiling water to be cooked as a satisfying side dish, a wonderful main course combined with veggies and a source

*Your salad will look like it belongs on the cover of a gourmet magazine and you'll look like a gastronomic genius.*

of protein, or added to soups and salads to provide variety, taste and texture. Because these foods are starchy and for many people can be consumed in large quantities as comfort foods, be aware of portion sizes. One cup cooked is generally equivalent to two starch servings and can be extended with a serving or two of vegetables.

## Low-calorie Italian salad dressing

Sometimes the taste of bottled fat-free or low-fat salad dressings can be disappointing. And even when they are fat-free, these dressings can still provide plenty of calories. There are exceptions of course. If you find one that you like, use it in moderate amounts and enjoy. Or try a flavored vinegar or my low-fat vinaigrette which is always a hit.

*And even when they are fat-free, these dressings can still provide plenty of calories.*

One low-calorie or fat-free salad dressing which I do find extremely useful is Italian. I use it to marinate skinless chicken breasts before coating with cornflake crumbs and baking, to turn leftover pasta combined with a few veggies into pasta salad or on its own to add zing to a mixed green salad.

## Bottled pasta sauce

In a perfect world, we'd all be making our own pasta sauce. We'd use fresh tomatoes, onion, garlic, basil, oregano, salt and pepper simmered gently on the stove while somebody would serenade us from a gondola below the kitchen window. But you probably don't have the time and Pavarotti hasn't come by lately. If anything changes, by all means go ahead and make your own sauce from scratch.

When you are squeezed for time, use a bottled meatless sauce as a base. Add your own lean ground beef, diced chicken, veggie "ground beef" or fresh or frozen vegetables to make a delicious sauce that will be ready in no time. You can also use your bottled sauce for making lasagna. To keep fat and calories low, you can choose one of the light varieties available at the supermarket.

## Canned tomatoes

Canned tomatoes are really handy to add to sauces, soups and stews. I especially like canned ground tomatoes for making the sauce for my meatballs and for adding rich flavor and color to cabbage soup. Many of my recipes seem to use tomatoes in some form or another, probably for two reasons. One, I love the taste and texture of tomatoes; and two, the phytochemical, lycopene that is found in tomatoes is believed to reduce the risk of cancer, especially prostate. No matter how you say it, "tomaito" or "tomahto", it's one healthy choice.

For those following a sodium restricted diet or who just want to reduce their salt intake, ground tomatoes with no added salt can be substituted in most recipes calling for regular canned tomatoes.

## Egg whites in a carton

Egg whites in a carton are terrific! You can use them to make deliciously light omelettes and frittatas, and in cooking and baking to reduce fat and cholesterol. By eliminating the step of cracking and separating whole eggs, they're not only convenient, they also remove the dilemma of what to do with the yolks. You won't have to feel guilty for throwing them out or feeding them to the dog.

Egg whites in a carton have been a staple in my refrigerator since they became available. Many of my clients who are achieving and maintaining their weight goals enjoy an egg white dish for breakfast, lunch or dinner, a few times a week.

The secret to cooking successfully with egg whites is to go "low and slow". Cook your egg whites in a non-stick pan sprayed with cooking spray, slowly on medium-low heat. Because they are fat-free, they need to be cooked carefully. Another method is to cook them covered in the microwave. Like my clients, you'll get used to the light white color and won't miss the look of whole eggs. Or you can add a pinch of turmeric for a golden touch of color.

Generally, 2 tbsp of egg whites in a carton is equivalent to 1 fresh egg white. ¼ cup of egg whites can be substituted for 1 whole egg in many recipes calling for whole eggs. ½ cup of egg whites is equivalent to 4 egg whites. Keep refrigerated, check expiry date and use within 7 days of opening to ensure freshness. Use this handy guide when you use egg whites in cartons.

*The secret to cooking successfully with egg whites is to go "low and slow".*

| Egg Whites in a Carton | Egg Whites |
|---|---|
| 2 tbsp (25 mL) | 1 egg white |
| ¼ cup (50 mL) | 2 egg whites |
| | 1 whole egg in recipes |
| ½ cup (125 mL) | 4 egg whites |
| 1 cup (250 mL) | 8 egg whites |

## Flavored vinegars

I'll never forget my first bottle of balsamic vinegar. It was given to me as a hostess gift. I had never seen balsamic vinegar before. After one taste, I was hooked. I couldn't believe how delicious it was. I splashed it liberally on our salad greens and within a week it was all gone.

When I went to the store to buy some more, imagine my surprise when I discovered that this wonderful vinegar was like a fine wine with a price-tag to match. I bought a much less expensive bottle as a replacement and have enjoyed it ever since.

Balsamic vinegar can be used by itself as a dressing or combined with a little olive oil. During BBQ season, I use it as a fat-free baste for grilling vegetables and chicken. Because of its natural sweetness, balsamic vinegar does provide calories, about 16 per tablespoon.

Another excellent vinegar that works well on its own is rice vinegar. I especially enjoy seasoned rice vinegar, which has a little added salt and sugar and provides about 20 calories per tablespoon. Other terrific vinegars include wine, cider, cranberry and champagne. Experiment, have fun and find one that can become your favorite too.

## Cooking spray

I probably should have mentioned this staple first as it is so basic to lighter food preparation. It makes almost any cooking surface non-stick without adding significant fat and calories.

*Vegetable cooking sprays now come in regular, olive oil and butter flavors.*

Cooking spray can be used to lightly spray a variety of foods like potato strips before you oven "fry" them, skinless chicken breasts and fish fillets before grilling to prevent them from sticking, and bagel rounds before oven toasting. And to make life more interesting, vegetable cooking sprays now come in regular, olive oil and butter flavors.

## Condiments, soup mixes

Other staples to add flavor to your cooking include condiments like mustards, ketchup, Worcestershire sauce, light soy and teriyaki sauces. These are all salty, so use them in moderation and add little, if any salt to your recipe.

Keep low-sodium chicken, vegetable and beef-flavored soup mixes on hand to use as a base for soups. Fat-free canned chicken soup can also be used as a stock. You can dilute the soup with extra water to cut down on salt.

## How to Lighten Up a Recipe

| Typical Lasagna Recipe Ingredients: | To Lighten Up Use: | Approx. Fat Saved (g) |
|---|---|---|
| 2 tbsp (25 mL) olive oil | olive oil cooking spray | 26 |
| 9 lasagna noodles | 9 lasagna noodles | - |
| 3 cups (750 mL) meat sauce | 3 cups (750 mL) meatless sauce | 24 |
| 1 lb (500 g) | ½ lb (250 g) | |
| Mozzarella cheese | part-skim Mozzarella cheese | 56 |
| 3 cups (750 mL) ricotta cheese, | 2 cups (500 mL)1% cottage cheese, | 90 |
| mixed with 2 eggs | mixed with 4 egg whites | 10 |
| 1 cup (250 mL) grated Parmesan cheese | ½ cup (125 mL) low-fat grated Parmesan cheese | 16 |
| | Total Fat Saved Per Recipe: | 222 g 1998 calories |
| | Total Fat Saved Per Serving (8 servings per recipe): | 28 g 250 calories |

You can see that we've reduced the amount of fat and many of the calories in this recipe by using lower fat alternatives and by cutting down on the quantity of cheese. In fact, 28 grams of fat is almost half the recommended daily intake of fat for a woman, one-third the daily intake of fat for a man. By saving 250 calories each day, you could reduce your weight by half a pound per week.

To make up for the reduced quantity of cheese, you can add a layer of fresh vegetables like sliced zucchini, mushrooms, spinach, onion, or red or green pepper.

Use the Lighten Up tool in Part 3 to reduce the fat and calories in some of the recipes that you're using now.

# CHAPTER 8

# Be a Social-Light

I T'S TIME to spread your wings. Now that you're seeing the light when eating at home with your enlightened cooking techniques and can't miss snack strategy, let's talk about how you can ease up on the fat and calories when you're eating out.

For most of my clients, eating out is part of their regular routine. It's likely a part of your busy lifestyle too. Whether it's for business, entertaining, socializing or grabbing a quick bite on the go, many people find themselves eating at least one meal a day or more away from home.

You can eat out and achieve and maintain your health and weight goals too. In fact, eating out in a healthy way can sometimes be easier than when you're eating at home. You're not tempted to go for second helpings and you're not nibbling while cooking or clearing the dishes. To eat like a social-light, all it takes is a few well-planned strategies before you hit the road.

*You're not tempted to go for second helpings and you're not nibbling while cooking or clearing the dishes.*

## Variety Rules

Choose a restaurant that serves a variety of food. Look for lower fat choices on the menu like salads (ask for the dressing on the side), grilled chicken and fish, egg white omelettes, and pastas available in smaller portion sizes.

Avoid a restaurant with a limited menu. By that I mean skip the local fish and chips hang-out or the burger shack. It will be almost impossible to see the light if all the food is fried and high in fat.

Instead, look for a restaurant with plenty of variety. You'll have an easier time. Some restaurants even highlight (pardon the pun) lighter choices on their menus and provide calorie and fat information. Be sure to let the manager know how much you appreciate this service. Make a list of favorite restaurants where you've enjoyed lighter meals. Suggest these restaurants when your friends ask you where you'd like to go out to eat.

*Look for a restaurant with plenty of variety. You'll have an easier time.*

## On the Menu

When you read a menu, look for the lighter items that will help you achieve your goals, instead of looking for something that's tempting but loaded with fat and calories. The grilled chicken breast, baked potato and salad with dressing on the side will be all the more satisfying knowing that you won't be sabotaging your healthy eating goal.

Key words and terms to look for are grilled, baked, steamed, poached, roasted, broiled, tomato sauce and broth. High-fat giveaways include fried, buttery, creamy, crispy, sautéed, cheesy, casserole and au gratin. Be sure to specify that grilled and broiled foods be prepared with as little fat as possible.

## Ask Questions

With your sweetest smile and assertive tone, ask your server to describe how the food is prepared and what comes with your entrée. Request that dressings and sauces be served on the side and that food be cooked with a minimum of fat. That way there will be no surprises. Don't be afraid to speak up just because you don't want to draw attention to yourself because you're eating in a healthy way.

This also applies if your food arrives other than the way you ordered it. Too often we will accept and eat food that we're not happy with. For example, a client told me that when she was out for dinner one evening, the fish that she had ordered grilled without fat came swimming in butter. She ate it anyway because she didn't want to make a fuss by sending it back. She didn't enjoy her meal because she was unused to the coated mouth-feel of the butter and she was unhappy about all the extra fat and calories that she had consumed.

Remember, you have the right to have it your way when you're paying the tab as long as your requests are reasonable and communicated in a courteous way. Most restaurants and staff are very accommodating. Low-fat requests are very common. I believe most restaurants really do try their best to please their patrons. If not, choose a restaurant that does.

## Pamper Yourself

Turn eating out into a "spa" experience. Treat yourself by having your food prepared for you by a professional chef, cooked to your specifications and served by attentive staff. Enjoy the restaurant event as a kind of pampering, rather than as an opportunity to indulge in higher fat and calorie-laden foods.

In the same way, you don't have to go to a real spa to enjoy a healthy vacation. If you're travelling by plane, order a low-fat meal for the flight when you make your reservation. While on holiday, take advantage of having time for yourself to do something active every day. Use the spa eating strategy when dining in restaurants. Being away from home doesn't mean that you have to pack on the pounds just because you've packed your bags.

*While on holiday, take advantage of having time for yourself to do something active every day.*

## Eating Around

*In North America, you can savor the tastes and flavors of exotic cultures without ever leaving home.*

In North America, you can savor the tastes and flavors of exotic cultures without ever leaving home. Greek, Chinese, Japanese, Italian, Thai, French, Mexican and Indian are just some of the fabulous cuisines from which to choose.

Added to these are neighbourhood delis that offer an endless array of choices. Steak houses again are all the rage. "All you can eat" buffets and fast food outlets seem to be everywhere you go. How can you eat your way around the world without having a waistline to match? A little careful planning and knowing what to order can make all the difference.

## Greece Doesn't Have to Mean Grease

Greek food is usually prepared with plenty of olive oil. In authentic Greek cuisine, olive oil is used liberally to preserve food and enhance flavor. It's the main source of fat in the Greek diet and may play a role in the low rate of heart disease in Mediterranean countries. Olives and olive oil have always been considered a precious commodity in Greece. Their consumption goes back to antiquity.

Having said all this about the fine points of olive oil, remember that olive oil is still a fat and fat is fattening. So your best picks at a Greek restaurant are a Greek salad with just a little feta cheese and a squirt of lemon juice, a chicken souvlaki (skewer) with rice, pita and a dab of tzatziki (yogurt dip). Higher fat choices are the lamb dishes, hummus, eggplant dips and roasted potatoes. Choose these less often.

## Use Your Noodle when You Eat Chinese

If we ate Chinese food in North America the way the Chinese do in China, we wouldn't have a problem with consuming too much fat and too many calories. In China, the main event is a small rice bowl accompanied by morsels of steamed or stir-fried fish, seafood, or pork with vegetables.

Compare this to a North American scenario—fried egg rolls and spring rolls, battered and fried sweet and sour chicken and shrimp, spare ribs, fried rice and Chinese noodles are typical fare. Instead go for lighter choices like consommé or Chinese vegetable soup, steamed rice and lightly stir-fried or steamed dishes that contain more vegetables than meat. If you tend to eat too quickly, ask for chopsticks to help you slow down.

*If you tend to eat too quickly, ask for chopsticks to help you slow down.*

To reduce sodium, ask that your food be prepared with no MSG (monosodium glutamate). Use condiments like plum sauce or mustard instead of soy sauce. Sip a steaming cup of green tea with your meal. Soon you won't need a fortune cookie to tell you that you're well on your way to achieving your healthy eating goals.

## Japanese Food—A Rice Way to Eat

Japanese food generally offers a wide array of healthy choices, although be careful as many can be high in salt. Teriyaki dishes, fish and vegetable sushi, steamed rice and miso soup are safe bets. Avoid deep-fried tempura. To keep from going overboard on the number of pieces of sushi you eat, start with a salad and miso soup.

At the cooking table, be sure to let your chef know in advance how you would like your food cooked. Ask for a minimum of oil on the grill, chicken without skin, seafood like shrimp, scallops and lobster without butter and beef lean and well-trimmed. Vegetarian entrées are also available. To be on the safe side, be sure to let your chef know your special requests before the meat cleavers and pepper mills start flying.

## Italian—Basta with the Pasta

"Basta (Italian for "enough") with the Pasta!" roared the headline when the story broke that we're overdoing it with pasta. It seems that North Americans had wishfully been believing that because this starchy food is low in fat, it was okay to consume heaping portion sizes and still stay trim.

Lighter choices at your favorite trattoria include grilled fish or chicken prepared with a minimum of oil, veal prepared in a wine sauce (not breaded and fried) or a small serving of pasta with chicken or seafood in a tomato-based Marinara sauce. As with Greek food, olive oil rules, so be sure to order your food with a minimum of oil.

*As with Greek food, olive oil rules, so be sure to order your food with a minimum of oil.*

Start your meal with a mixed salad with vinaigrette dressing on the side or a minestrone soup. If you want pasta for a main course, by all means, have it. Just ask for an appetizer-size portion.

Resist the temptation to soak your bread in the olive oil which is often put on the table instead of butter. Instead, feel free to enjoy a few dabs with a slice of crusty bread. Just be sure to count the bread and oil as part of your starch and fat for the meal. For dessert, some fresh berries and a decaf cappuccino made with low-fat milk combine to make the perfect finale to a light and satisfying meal. You'll be singing "That's Amore!" in no time.

## Thai One On

I've learned about Thai cuisine, richly perfumed with lemon grass, coriander and spices, from one of my clients. I often see Thai spring rolls on the food diaries he so faithfully keeps for me. Before I can raise an eyebrow, he always assures me that these rolls are actually raw veggies wrapped in a soft rice paper and are definitely not fried.

Other lower fat options he enjoys on the Thai menu include grilled satays (skewers of grilled chicken or beef) without the peanut sauce, Pad thai, steamed or grilled fish, stir-fry dishes prepared with a minimum of oil and most salads served with dressing on the side. To be avoided, he points out, are the deep-fried choices and dishes prepared with coconut milk or cream. A very savvy client indeed.

## La Belle Nouvelle

French cuisine is known for its liberal use of butter and cream, often found in sauces like hollandaise, bearnaise and bechamel. A good rule of thumb in French and in fact in most restaurants, is to request that these sauces and all dressings be served separately on the side. That way, you can decide how much you will have. Lighter sauces are the wine-based Bordelaise and the tomato-based Provençale.

With Nouvelle cuisine, the portions aren't very large, so you shouldn't have a problem when it comes to serving sizes. A grilled meat, fish or poultry entrée is usually a good choice with a simply cooked vegetable and potato instead of "frites" which are fried. Consommé soup or green salad are low-fat starters.

Avoid French onion soup which is usually topped with a layer of cheese. Pass on the au gratin dishes that are prepared with buttered crumbs and cheese. French chefs generally serve smaller starchy side dishes, so treat yourself to a slice or two of the crusty French baguette. Just skip the butter. For dessert, go for some fresh berries (without the creme fraiche) and a "skinny" cafe au lait made with skim milk.

*With Nouvelle cuisine, the portions aren't very large, so you shouldn't have a problem when it comes to serving sizes.*

## South of the Border, Down Mexico Weigh

Mexican food is generally high in fat as many items are either deep fried or served with cheese, sour cream and higher fat dips like guacamole. Dishes often include refried beans, generally made with lard.

To keep fat and calories in line, choose a garden salad as an appetizer instead of fried nacho chips. For a main course, opt for a soft taco or burrito filled with grilled chicken, lean beef and vegetables. Avoid the higher fat toppings and load up on chopped tomatoes, shredded lettuce and sliced onions instead. Other good choices are mixed bean salads and chili, but be sure to ask a few questions about the fat content. Remember, planning ahead means no surprises, Amigo.

## Indian—Ghee Wiz

Indian food offers a dazzling array of flavors, textures and colors. The abundant use of spices, vegetables, salads, yogurt, lean chicken and fish, lentils and vegetarian options ensure that healthy choices can be made. A yogurt-based curry dish is often a good choice. So is the beautiful ruby red Tandoori chicken.

*The main caution with Indian food, is that much of the food is prepared with ghee, also known as clarified butter.*

Enjoy your meal with plain rice or naan, a pita-type Indian flatbread which is low in fat. The main caution with Indian food, is that much of the food is prepared with ghee, also known as clarified butter. Ask that your food be prepared without ghee and avoid dishes where it is used.

## Deli De-lites

Kishka, corned beef, blintzes and latkes are just a few of the higher fat delicacies you'll find at your local smoked meat emporium. They're all right up there on the high-fat Richter scale, probably because their roots are in Eastern Europe. This was a mainly agrarian society. A high-fat diet would ensure plenty of calories needed for working in the fields. Since most of us here in North America want to avoid consuming excess calories and fat, we'll have to lighten up when we opt for deli food.

Lighter choices include lean pastrami, roast beef or turkey breast sandwiches, regular (not creamy) coleslaw, dill pickles, chicken soup with a few noodles (a matzo ball, occasionally), boiled chicken in the pot (without the skin) and gefilte fish with horseradish. Go for rye bread or pumpernickel instead of challah, which is generally higher in fat and calories. A glass tea and a baked apple make a perfect ending. What could be bad? Enjoy!

## Steak House Fare

Steak houses are popular again with what seem like brontosaurus-size servings of steaks and ribs. Side-dishes like whole fried onions can pack about two thousand calories and over one hundred and fifty grams of fat with dipping sauce. They're bloomin' with fat and calories! Knowing how to manoeuvre on the menu can save the day.

*Steak houses are popular again with what seem like brontosaurus-size servings of steaks and ribs.*

Choose the smallest size steak on the menu, grilled or broiled without fat. Leaner cuts include filet mignon, sirloin and flank steak. Avoid the mega-size portions of rib and porterhouse steaks which really load on the fat and calories. If the restaurant sends their steaks out of the kitchen sizzling with a knob of butter on top, let them know ahead of time that you'll take a pass on the extra fat.

Start with a garden salad and choose a baked potato, without butter or sour cream and some steamed broccoli, if available. Skip the garlic bread. Instead ask for garlic toasted bread which is like garlic bread without the butter.

If a grilled chicken breast, fish or seafood is on the menu, you might want to choose one of these. If you haven't had beef all week, go for the steak. Just balance it later with some lighter choices. Following the Fab Four for choosing protein foods allows for guilt-free enjoyment of all your favorites while still being able to achieve and maintain your healthy eating goal.

## The Battle of the Buffet

An all-you-can-eat buffet can be a minefield of hidden fat and calories. In addition, it's natural to think that unless you eat enough for a whole week, you're not getting your money's worth. You're going to need a well-designed plan of attack to emerge victorious.

Think of the buffet as a visual menu, not an invitation to try one of everything on the table. Plan your attack. Start with reconnaissance. Review the entire selection on the buffet before you start filling your plate. Make a mental note of what you will choose for your main course or entrée.

Plan to make three trips to the buffet. The first is for your salad course, the second for your entrée and the third for dessert. This way you won't feel left out when those around you are making round-trips to refill their plates.

For your salad course, choose plain or undressed salads and vegetables, with dressing on the side. If salads are dressed, choose salads in a vinaigrette rather than a creamy dressing. Vinaigrettes don't cling to the leaves like creamy dressings do, so you'll get less dressing, fat and calories.

You can use this strategy when you visit a salad bar too. Remember, everything on the salad bar isn't necessarily low in fat and calories. So choose carefully. Fill your plate with undressed greens and vegetables.

Here's a neat trick. As a topping, you can add some veggies that are marinated in a vinaigrette. This can double as your salad dressing and will add lots of flavor to your salad. Add some chickpeas or cottage cheese for protein, a whole grain roll and you're all set.

Back to the buffet. For your main course, keep the portion of meat, fish or poultry to about three ounces (100 g) or the size of a small deck of cards. Choose baked, steamed or

*Think of the buffet as a visual menu, not an invitation to try one of everything on the table.*

grilled rather that fried. Fill your plate with cooked vegetables and a small portion of starch or a whole grain roll.

Whenever possible, ask for gravy or sauces on the side and use as little as possible. If the food is served from a large chafing dish, serve yourself from the top because gravies and sauces (with most of the fat) tend to sink to the bottom.

Season foods with fresh ground pepper instead of salt. For dessert, fill your plate with fresh fruit first. Have a small serving of your favorite dessert, if you wish.

## The Brunch Bunch

Many hotel dining rooms offer bountiful breakfast buffets daily or on the weekend. Ordering items from the menu often works out to be about the same price as ordering the full buffet breakfast, so most people opt for the buffet. Not the most economical move nutritionally, because you often end up paying the price in terms of unwanted fat and calories.

You can use the three-trip strategy for a breakfast buffet, especially if it's on the weekend and your breakfast becomes brunch. Your first trip can be for some hot or cold cereal with skim milk, the second for a pancake or two or an egg white dish made with minimal fat, and the third for fresh fruit with a topping of low-fat yogurt.

*You can use the three-trip strategy for a breakfast buffet, especially if it's on the weekend and your breakfast becomes brunch.*

This is still an ample breakfast but it is lower in fat and calories than the traditional one of juice, scrambled eggs, French toast, bacon, sausage, fried potatoes, muffins and sweet rolls.

When you do order à la carte, fresh fruit with low-fat yogurt, hot or cold cereal with low-fat milk, whole wheat toast or an English muffin with jam, or an egg white dish are all healthy choices.

## Life in the Fast Lane

You probably think that fast food is on your list of no-no's. Since you're living in the real world, let's be realistic. In your line of work, you may spend a great deal of time in your car. Or you may have to grab a quick meal with your kids before appointments and activities. You may have little choice but to eat some fast food from time to time.

Fast food restaurants now offer lighter, healthier options like soups, salad bars, grilled chicken sandwiches and wraps, baked potatoes, juices and low-fat milk. With so many healthy choices, a meal at a fast food outlet doesn't have to be a double burger with cheese, fries and a milkshake.

*With so many healthy choices, a meal at a fast food outlet doesn't have t o be a double burger with cheese, fries and a milkshake.*

Instead, go for a small regular burger or grilled chicken sandwich (hold the mayo), vegetable soup, salad or baked potato if it's offered and a juice or sugar-free soft drink. Avoid the fried chicken or fish sandwiches which often have more fat than the burger. This may be news to some of you, but it's true.

I know the regular burger tends to look kiddie size. That's because we've all grown accustomed to the super-size food portions served in restaurants these days. The regular burger is probably all your body really needs.

For a fast food breakfast choose pancakes with a little syrup, or an English muffin with a bit of jam, low-fat milk or juice. Skip the scrambled eggs, breakfast meats, fried potatoes, donuts, croissants, Danish and jumbo-muffins which I call "the lumberjack" breakfast.

To sit in your car driving the kids to school, to do errands, to work at your desk or computer, talk on the phone or sit in meetings most of the morning, you don't need the mega-calories to last you until lunch. See the light at breakfast and the rest of the day will follow.

# Social-Lighting

There's no need to panic over your next dinner party invitation now that you've started seeing the light. I've learned a very clever strategy from Norman the "Nutritionist" to avoid overeating at someone's home. Of course, he didn't realize he was teaching me anything at all. He was just being himself.

I always know when Norman's not hungry at meal-time. That's when the compliments and raves about the food start flowing. "That chicken looks fabulous" really means, "I had a big lunch and I'm not very hungry." "What a beautiful-looking stew" means, "I'll be doing more looking than eating at this meal".

Sometimes he uses the "stall" technique. "I'll just wait until it cools off." This of course means, "Maybe by then you won't notice that I'm not going to have any."

So when you're at a dinner party and you don't want to overeat, take a tip from Norman the "Nutritionist." Compliment lavishly and eat lightly. Your host or hostess will be happy that you're enjoying yourself and won't have to measure your pleasure with how much you eat.

If your host or hostess is very persistent, you might have to use the stall method. It works every time!

# Holiday Eating Strategy

Whether it's Thanksgiving, Christmas, Chanukah, New Year's, Easter or Passover, you can survive holiday eating feeling confident, relaxed, trim, and healthy. The following tips will show you how.

### Never arrive at a party too hungry.

When you arrive at a party famished, you head straight for the cocktail weenies and the chip dip. You may find yourself devouring foods that you don't even like. To avoid temptation,

*When you arrive at a party famished, you head straight for the cocktail weenies and the chip dip.*

enjoy a light snack before you go. Your snack will take the edge off your hunger. The fried finger foods will be much easier to resist. You'll probably have a better time as you eat sensibly and enjoy the food you choose.

## Offer to bring your host or hostess a salad or fresh fruit platter.

Bring a salad with a light vinaigrette, veggies with yogurt dip or cut-up fresh fruit platter. These tend to be time-consuming to prepare. Your thoughtfulness will be appreciated and you'll be assured that there will be some healthy choices for you to eat too.

## Keep a safe distance from the buffet table.

When it's time to eat, don't be the first person at the buffet. Check out what's on the table before you start filling your plate. Plan ahead and be selective. Choose moderate portions of your holiday favorites.

After you've made your choices, stay a safe distance from the food table. Often just the sight of food can be a trigger to overeat. As the cliché goes, "out of sight, out of mind". Sip a mineral water, talk to your pals or do some dancing. It will definitely take your mind off the cheese balls.

## Mineral water, a sugar-free soft drink or tomato juice on ice are great party drinks.

As long as you have one of these drinks in your hand, you'll be less tempted or coaxed to have an alcohol-containing beverage. This is a great strategy to help you maintain a moderate intake of alcohol. One drink is equivalent to 5 oz/150 mL of wine, 12 oz/350 mL of beer or 1½ oz/50 mL of liquor.

## When the party is at your place, send your guests home with doggie bags.

Pack up leftovers and send them home with your guests. If you still have food left over, you probably prepared too much. Get your family and friends to help store the leftovers, preferably in the freezer. That way, the goodies will be less handy for nibbling.

Be sure to make some notes for next time, so you'll prepare less. This may help to avoid some of the extra work, expense and temptation for future get-togethers.

## Drink lots of water.

Extra water, at least 8 cups a day, will help keep you well-hydrated. Salty foods and alcoholic beverages increase your need for water.

## Maintain your regular meals and snacks, activity, sleep and rest as best you can.

Holidays aren't times when you have to put all your healthy habits on hold. Even if you can't keep to your usual healthy eating routine, every bit helps. Healthy eating and living are a continuum of choices. Balance and moderation replace all or nothing. This approach will help you achieve and maintain your healthy lifestyle goals, once and for all.

*Healthy eating and living are a continuum of choices. Balance and moderation replace all or nothing.*

# Ten Healthy Host Or Hostess Gifts

When you're invited to someone's house, are you stumped about what to bring as a gift? Now that you're seeing the light, skip the box of candy or cookies. Instead, share the wealth of health. Give a gift that promotes pleasure and healthy living. Any one of these will surely be treasured.

### 1. mustards, salsa, fruit spreads

Fill a small basket available at craft stores, with an assortment of mustards, salsa or fruit spreads. Wrap the basket in festive tissue paper and tie with a pretty ribbon. This makes a creative and less expensive alternative to ready-made gift baskets.

### 2. flavored vinegar

Balsamic vinegar is always wonderful, but other delicious and interesting herb and fruit varieties are also available. I recently received a stunning bottle of cranberry vinegar which is on display in my kitchen. I can't wait to taste it!

### 3. cold-pressed extra-virgin olive oil

Anything this special will be savored in tiny amounts. Give this healthful oil to be enjoyed by the light-hearted.

### 4. a collection of serviettes, party plates, festive tumblers

These are always welcome, especially for special holidays or BBQ season.

### 5. a medley of herbs and spices

*In summer give an assortment of steak spice, peppercorns, dill and cilantro.*

A great way to add zing to festive and everyday cooking is with the artful use of herbs and spices. Fill a flower pot in summer, a wicker basket in spring or an evergreen-trimmed box in winter with a medley of spices and herbs on a seasonal theme. In summer give an assortment of steak spice, peppercorns, dill and cilantro. In the fall, switch to sage, rosemary, and thyme. At Christmas, nutmeg, cinnamon sticks, ginger and allspice are always welcome.

## 6. yogurt cheese herb dip

Bring along an assortment of veggies with a fat-free yogurt cheese dip. Place on a new acrylic or glass serving platter that can be kept and enjoyed after the party's over.

## 7. chocolate meringues

Satisfying even to the most ardent chocoholic, these crispy fat-free delights make a lovely gift packed in a decorative tin.

## 8. a gift tray of assorted dried fruit

Dried fruits are a good source of iron, fiber and potassium. And they're always a welcome addition to a dessert table. Make your own assortment by arranging a few kinds of dried fruits like apricots, dates, dried figs, pitted prunes or giant raisins on a wicker tray, cover with colored cellophane wrap, and decorate with festive ribbon and a bow.

## 9. a dozen low-fat muffins

When you're invited for tea, coffee or brunch, offer to make a dozen low-fat muffins. Pack them in a fabric-covered box. Add a few chocolate chips to each muffin before baking to add the richness of chocolate without a lot of extra fat and calories.

## 10. an assortment of herbal teas

What better way to relax and unwind after all the guests have gone? Fill a mug or small ceramic teapot with a variety of herbal teas like camomile, peppermint and rosehip for a gift that says "Relax and enjoy. You deserve it."

*"Relax and enjoy. You deserve it."*

# BBQ ABC's

One of the joys of summertime is eating food cooked outdoors over an open grill. Keep your food healthy by preventing meat fat from dripping onto wood, charcoal or gas flames. This can form potentially cancer-causing chemicals.

These chemicals can be deposited on food by rising smoke or flare-ups and whenever meat is cooked until charred or burnt. Avoid being a five-alarm chef and follow these simple precautions to make sure that your food is both safe and delicious to eat.

1. Choose meats well-trimmed of all visible fat and remove skin from poultry before grilling.

2. Marinate meats and poultry to reduce the potential for cancer-causing chemicals.

3. Raise the grill well above the coals or flame. Avoid placing meat directly over the coals so you can prevent fat dripping onto them.

4. To reduce grilling time, partially precook meat in the microwave or oven, then finish on the grill.

5. Wrap food with foil to reduce direct contact with smoke or flames, or place a metal pan between the meat and the coals to catch the dripping fat.

6. Remove meat briefly or reduce heat if dripping fat creates a lot of smoke.

7. Avoid eating charred parts of the food.

8. Always discard marinades that have been used for raw meats and poultry. Place cooked foods on clean plates only.

9. Be sure to thoroughly cook burgers made from ground meat or poultry to destroy potentially harmful bacteria. These bacteria generally live on the surface of meats and are destroyed by high heat during cooking. When meat is ground however, these surface bacteria can be mixed in throughout the meat mixture. They will only be destroyed if the burger is thoroughly cooked and no longer pink inside.

10. Alternate BBQ'ing with other cooking methods like steaming, broiling and stir-frying. Remember, variety rules.

# CHAPTER 9

# Light on Your Feet

BEING SEDENTARY is hazardous to your health, not to mention your waistline. So it's time to get moving.

Now I can just see some of you shaking your heads and saying "no way". You'd probably rather have a tooth drilled instead. (And we all know how much fun that is!) I can still remember how painfully self-conscious I was about my over-weight body in my high-school gym uniform with the leg bands digging into my thighs.

In fact, before I joined The Fitness Institute, I was intim-idated about walking through the front door. I had visions of bodies beautiful romping around in form-fitting workout wear, flexing muscles and showing off washboard stomachs. How could I possibly fit in, me, who had never exercised before?

When I finally did get up the courage to go, I was relieved to find myself in a warm, friendly and supportive environment. I saw people of all ages, shapes and sizes. They shared a common goal of getting their bodies moving and improving their health and well-being. I had no trouble fit-ting in, because that's what I wanted too. That was my first lesson in fitness. It's for everybody and every body.

*That was my first lesson in fitness. It's for everybody and every body.*

Did you know that you need to decrease your intake by 3500 calories to reduce your body weight by one pound? You can do this by eating less fat and fewer calories so your body will dip into its own fat reserves for fuel.

But what if I told you that you could give this process a boost by burning some extra calories and revving up your metabolism at the same time? I thought you'd be interested. Well, that's exactly what exercise does.

Like I did, I know some of you are cringeing just at the mention of the word "exercise". I can't blame you. That's because you're thinking that exercise has to happen in a gym, it makes you sweat, it's a lot of work and it bores you to tears. I have a good idea. Instead of "exercise", from now on, we'll call it "activity". Activity is anything that gets you moving. You can even have fun doing it. From walking to roller-blading to gardening to playing catch with your kids, as long as you "just do it" like the ad says, you're being active and achieving your goals.

When I joined The Fitness Institute, I loved the aerobics classes. I'd buy myself a new workout leotard every so often that made me feel like I was "Wonder Woman." And as a stay-at-home young mother I enjoyed being in a group class with other women. The fun of dancing to upbeat music made my workout especially enjoyable. It was perfect for me because it suited my "workout personality".

I much preferred it to wearing a baggy T-shirt and riding a stationary bicycle in the gym. To this day, my favorite workout is still a class at The Fitness Institute. But that's me. Everyone has their own workout personality. Getting to know yours will help you find the activity that you enjoy. And guess what? When you find an activity you enjoy, you'll keep doing it. And that's the best there is. One that you enjoy and that you keep doing.

*Like I did, I know some of you are cringeing just at the mention of the word "exercise".*

Thankfully, we're all different. Some folks are limited in time and like to do things at their own pace. For them, popping a workout tape into the VCR (and there's no need to get bored, the variety is endless), walking on a treadmill at home, or having a personalized program that they can do whenever they get to the gym will be ideal.

Some, like Norman the "Nutritionist," love the outdoors and like to jog or walk, rain or shine. One of my clients has taken up birding. She gets to go hiking with like-minded enthusiasts and to enjoy the wonders of nature at the same time. What could be better? Everyone's idea of a workout is different and that's just fine. Get to know yours. Doing it is what counts.

*Everyone's idea of a workout is different and that's just fine.*

Which brings me to my next point. People often want to know what the best fat-burning exercise is. You already know the answer. It's the one that you enjoy because that's the one you'll do. And the doing is everything.

Theoretically, the best fat or calorie-burner might be cross-country skiing, but if you live in the city, or if it's summer and you don't have access to a cross-country skiing machine, you're not doing it. So it makes no difference if it's a great fat-burner or not.

There are lots of other ways to be physically active that have nothing to do with working out. Simple moves like parking your car a little further from your destination, walking instead of driving to the mailbox to post a letter, climbing up a few flights of stairs instead of taking the elevator (doctors do this all the time in hospitals to keep in shape), going dancing on the weekend instead of to a movie or out for dinner, playing ball with your kids, raking leaves or joining a mall walking group for an early morning get-together with friends, are all ways to move, burn calories and be more physically active.

I know I seem to be emphasizing the calorie-burning benefits of being physically active. There are many other benefits from being active that are just as important, maybe even more important. Regular physical activity can help reduce mild anxiety and depression, strengthen bones and help prevent osteoporosis, reduce stress, increase strength and flexibility, reduce blood pressure, improve blood sugar control, prevent cardiovascular disease and even slow the ageing process. If we could bottle it, we'd be taking one a day.

In fact, that's not a bad idea! Aim to be physically active every single day. Whether it's walking around the block before dinner, doing sit-ups while watching TV, or doing a full workout at the gym, just do it, do it, do it. You'll be glad you did.

## How to Get Started

1. Check with your doctor before increasing your physical activity or starting any new fitness program.

*Check with your doctor before increasing your physical activity or starting any new fitness program.*

2. Choose activities that suit your workout personality and lifestyle. Do you like group activities like step aerobic classes, competitive sports like racquetball or baseball, or solo programs that you can do in the gym or at home? The answers to these questions will help determine what will be best for you.

3. Set realistic goals. Think about your daily routine. At what points in the day could you increase your activity? If weekdays are really hectic, what about the weekend?

4. If you've never belonged to a fitness club, ask if they offer a trial membership so you can realistically assess if you'll like it. This way, you won't end up wasting a lot of money if you don't use your membership.

5. Beginners should consider group activities like low-impact aerobics classes (done in the gym or in the pool as aquabics) or even walking with a buddy, which can be more motivating than going it alone.

## A Word about Walking

Walking is one of the easiest ways to get physically active. Here are a few tips to get the most from your walking program.

1. Invest in a good pair of walking shoes. The support they provide will be well worth the cost.

2. Always stretch your calves, shins and thighs before and after your walk. This is very important to avoid pain or injury. Hold each stretch for a minimum of 30 seconds. Never, ever bounce.

3. Start slowly. Work up your speed and distance gradually.

4. An appropriate walking pace is one at which you are able to chat comfortably to workout pals without getting out of breath.

5. Dress suitably when walking out of doors. A good idea is layers that can be removed as your body warms up. Wear protective sun block and a hat, especially on sunny days.

6. Drink plenty of water before, during and after any form of physical activity.

*Drink plenty of water before, during and after any form of physical activity.*

## Take a FITT

The FITT Principle is a useful guide to help establish realistic goals for a workout routine. I have "lightened up" these guidelines to provide some tips for any couch potatoes like I was, who may be reading this.

**F** - frequency - ideally 3 to 5 times a week or more, or just more than you're doing now.

**I** - intensity - 60% to 85% of your maximum heart rate, or more energy that it takes to change channels with the TV remote.

**T** - type of activity - one that you enjoy, and if you can't think of one, that may be part of the problem. P.S. Start with a short walk with a buddy, which is always fun.

**T** - time - at least 10-20 minutes of continuous activity, or longer than it takes to walk from the den to the refrigerator to get a snack.

## Your Workout Personality

It's important to match your workout to your personality. Psychologists say the reason people dislike working out is they haven't chosen an activity that really suits them. Read these workout personality profiles and then do the self-assessment quiz found in Part 3. It will help you determine your workout personality so you can identify activities that you'll enjoy.

*Psychologists say the reason people dislike working out is they haven't chosen an activity that really suits them.*

## Workout Personality Profiles

**Solo Type:** You like doing your own thing. You enjoy outdoor activities like walking, jogging, skating, cross-country skiing, or bicycling. Indoors, you prefer treadmill walking, stationary bicycling, stair-climbing, swimming lengths in the pool or working out with weights.

**Social Type:** There's more fun in numbers for you. You enjoy group classes and showing off a new workout outfit every now and then. You probably like dance classes, step aerobics, water fitness classes, spinning, yoga, and stretch and strength classes.

**Competitive Type:** You're after a challenge. You need a game or a match to get you moving. A game of squash, racquetball, tennis, baseball, basketball, ping-pong, volleyball, or anything you can do while humming the theme from Rocky is right for you.

**Cross-trainer Type:** You'll never get bored with your workout. You like a mix of activities, alone or in a group. An interval workout class or your own program suits you just fine, but so does an outdoors solo jog or walk finished off with a stint on weights in the gym.

*You'll never get bored with your workout. You like a mix of activities, alone or in a group.*

# CHAPTER 10

# De-light-ful Eating Plans

O NE OF THE MOST effective tools to help you achieve your goals is your national food guide. In Canada, it's Canada's Food Guide to Healthy Eating. In the U.S. it's the Food Guide Pyramid.

These food guides have been revised and updated to reflect current nutrition recommendations for healthy living.

If you're not familiar with the guides, they're not the four sectioned circle you may remember from health class. Canada's Food Guide looks like a colorful rainbow depicting a wide variety of foods to eat. You can get a copy of the guide from your local health unit, from Health Canada in Ottawa at (613) 954-5995 or on-line at http://www.hc-sc.gc.ca/hppb/nutrition.

The U.S. Food Guide Pyramid is, as the name suggests, a broad-based pyramid, with grains, vegetables and fruits as the foundation of a healthy diet. The Food Guide Pyramid can be obtained from your local public health nutritionist, from the Center for Nutrition Policy and Promotion in Washington, D.C. at (202) 606-8000 or on-line at http://www.usda.gov/cnpp.

The largest food group on both Canada's Food Guide and the Food Guide Pyramid is the grain products, then come the vegetables and fruit, followed by milk products and

*These food guides have been revised and updated to reflect current nutrition recommendations for healthy living.*

finally, meat and alternatives. The grains, along with the vegetables and fruit categories are the two largest food groups because they provide carbohydrate, your fuel, or what I call the gasoline that keeps your engine purring all day long.

The milk group provides important vitamins and minerals like calcium for healthy bones, a little carbohydrate (lactose) and protein for building blocks. The smallest group, meat and alternatives provides protein for more building blocks and important minerals like iron, zinc and magnesium.

One reason the latter two food groups are the smallest of the four is that they can contain saturated fat, the one that potentially raises serum cholesterol. Remember, you want to keep your intake of this fat to a minimum. A second reason is that these groups provide mostly protein. Protein is used mainly for building blocks, not for fuel, so your body needs these foods in smaller quantities.

One of the guides' key messages is to choose a variety of foods. You need about fifty nutrients or more each day for good health. By eating an assortment of foods, you have the best chance of getting them all.

Also, different foods have varying amounts of fat. Variety helps you balance your fat intake. Finally, variety ensures that your food intake won't become boring and you won't tire of your healthy way of eating.

A second key message is to choose lower fat foods more often. This is certainly in keeping with our seeing the light approach to healthy eating and healthy weights. I couldn't agree more.

The food guides recommend choosing whole and enriched grains and cereals to help ensure that you meet the recommended twenty-five to thirty-five grams of fiber each day, along with your daily dose of iron and B vitamins.

For vegetables and fruits, choose deep green and orange varieties more often because these are the most nutritious.

> *A second key message is to choose lower fat foods more often. This is certainly in keeping with our seeing the light approach to healthy eating and healthy weights.*

They're just bursting with beta-carotene, vitamin C and folate. Milk products should be low in fat, as should the choices from the meat and alternatives group. By alternatives, the guides mean dried peas, beans and lentils, and other protein sources like tofu and peanut butter.

These guides work beautifully for healthy eating, and for achieving and maintaining your healthy weight goals too. The other foods group includes foods that are generally higher in fat, sugar and calories. These foods should be eaten less often, but not banished from your life forever. Just remember the healthy eating continuum. Then all foods can fit.

*These guides work beautifully for healthy eating, and for achieving and maintaining your healthy weight goals too.*

## Different Strokes for Different Folks

You can use the suggested number of servings per day printed on the the food guides to design your healthy eating plan. A range is provided for each food group because people of different ages, sizes, sex and activity levels need different amounts of food. The following table shows the number of food servings per day suggested by both guides.

| Number of Food Servings Per Day | | | |
|---|---|---|---|
| A Rainbow of Choices<br>Canada's Food Guide to Healthy Eating | | Pyramid Power<br>The U.S. Food Guide Pyramid | |
| Grain Products | 5-12 | Bread, Cereal, Rice & Pasta | 6-11 |
| Vegetables and Fruit | 5-10 | Vegetables 3-5    Fruit | 2-4 |
| Milk Products | 2-4 | Milk, Yogurt & Cheese | 2-3 |
| Meat & Alternatives | 2-3 | Meat, Poultry, Fish, Dry Beans,<br>Eggs & Nuts | 2-3 |
| Other Foods - Use in moderation | | Fats, Oils & Sweets - Use Sparingly | |
| Source: Canada's Food Guide to Healthy Eating, Minister of Supply and Services Canada, 1992. | | Source: The Food Guide Pyramid, United States Department of Agriculture, 1992. | |

## The Guiding Light

Using the food guide, a relatively inactive woman wanting to reduce her weight might start with the lowest numbers suggested for each food group. This would give her five or six servings of grains, two vegetables and three fruits, two servings of milk products, and another two of meat and alternatives. To this, she could add three to four teaspoons of oil from the other foods for cooking or salads, and she's ready to go.

Depending on her personal preference and lifestyle, she might want to distribute her grains this way: one for breakfast, two for lunch, one for snack and one or two for dinner. She might have at least one vegetable each for lunch and dinner, and one fruit with or after each meal. She could also divide her meat and alternatives between lunch and dinner. One milk at breakfast and one for a snack completes her day. For balanced eating, it's a good idea to represent at least three of the four food groups at each meal.

If she is achieving her goal of 1-2 lbs (0.5–1.0 kg) of weight reduction per week and she is satisfied with this level of intake, she could continue following this basic eating plan until she achieves her healthy weight goal. At that point she could gradually increase the number of servings per food group so that she will maintain her weight instead of continuing to reduce.

A healthy eating plan for a more active woman or man would include more choices from each food group. The upper level of choices would be suitable for growing teens and/or very active individuals.

You may still be a little unsure of how to follow the guides to help you reduce your weight, so here are some sample menus to show you how.

*For balanced eating, it's a good idea to represent at least three of the four food groups at each meal.*

# Healthy Eating Plan I*

5 or 6 Grain Products
2 Vegetables (or more) and 3 Fruit
2 Milk Products

2 Meat and Alternatives
3-4 tsp Fats and Oils (Other Foods)

**Breakfast:**

| | |
|---|---|
| 1 Grain | 1 slice toast or 1 oz (30 g) cold unsweetened cereal or ¾ cup (175 mL) hot cereal |
| 1 Fruit | one medium orange or ½ cup (125 mL) berries |
| 1 Milk | 1 cup (250 mL) skim milk or ¾ cup (175 mL) fat-free yogurt |

**Lunch:**

| | |
|---|---|
| 2 Grain | 2 slices bread or 2 oz (50 g) bagel or roll |
| 1 Vegetable | 1 cup (250 mL) salad or vegetable soup |
| 1 Meat | 2-3 oz (50-100 g) turkey slices or ½ cup (125 mL) water-packed tuna |
| 1 Fat | 2 tsp (10 mL) low-fat mayo or 1 tbsp (15 mL) low-fat salad dressing or 1 tsp(5 mL) oil |

**Snack (afternoon or evening):**

| | |
|---|---|
| 1 Grain | 4 melba toast |
| 1 Fruit | ½ cup (125 mL) mixed fruit |
| 1 Milk | ¾ cup (175 mL) fat-free yogurt |

**Dinner:**

| | |
|---|---|
| 1-2 Grain | ½ cup (125 mL) - 1 cup (250 mL) rice or pasta or 1-2 slices bread |
| 1 Vegetable | ½ cup (125 mL) cooked broccoli |
| 1 Fruit | 1 baked apple |
| 1 Meat | 3 oz (100 g) lean poultry, meat or fish or ¾ cup (175 mL) beans or ⅓ cup (75 mL) tofu |
| 2-3 Fat | 2-3 tsp (10-15 mL) oil |

**Fats and Oils Choices (Other Foods):**
1 tsp (5 mL) oil, non-hydrogenated margarine or mayonnaise
2 tsp (10 mL) low-fat mayonnaise, cream cheese or peanut butter
1-2 tbsp (15-25 mL) low-fat salad dressing
6 olives

\* Serving sizes are per Canada's Food Guide to Healthy Eating. Check U.S. Food Guide Pyramid for corresponding serving sizes. This eating plan provides approximately 1200–1300 calories per day.

# Healthy Eating Plan II*

6 Grain Products
3 Vegetables (or more) and 4 Fruit
3 Milk Products

2 Meat and Alternatives
3-4 Fats and Oils (Other Foods)

**Breakfast:**

| | |
|---|---|
| 1 Grain | 1 slice toast or 1 oz (30 g) cold unsweetened cereal or ¾ cup (175 mL) hot cereal |
| 1 Fruit | one medium orange or ½ cup (125 mL) berries |
| 1 Milk | 1 cup (250 mL) skim milk or ¾ cup (175 mL) fat-free yogurt |

**Lunch:**

| | |
|---|---|
| 2 Grain | 2 slices bread or 2 oz (50g) bagel or roll |
| 1 Vegetable | 1 cup (250 mL) salad or vegetable soup |
| 1 Meat | 2-3 oz (50-100g) turkey slices or ½ cup water-packed tuna |
| 1 Fat | 2 tsp (10 mL) low-fat mayo or 1 tbsp (15 mL) low-fat salad dressing or 1 tsp (5 mL) oil |

**Snack (afternoon and evening):**

| | |
|---|---|
| 1 Grain | 4 melba toast |
| 1 Fruit | ½ cup (125 mL) mixed fruit |
| 1 Milk | ¾ cup (175 mL) fat-free yogurt |

**Dinner:**

| | |
|---|---|
| 1 Grain | ½ cup (125 mL) rice or pasta or 1 slice bread |
| 2 Vegetable | ½ cup (125 mL) cooked peas and ½ cup (125 mL) cooked broccoli |
| 1 Fruit | 1 baked apple |
| 1 Meat | 3 oz (100 g) lean poultry, meat or fish or ¾ cup (175 mL) beans or ⅓ cup (75 mL) tofu |
| 2-3 Fat | 2-3 tsp (10-15 mL) oil |

**Fats and Oils Choices (Other Foods):**

1 tsp (5 mL) oil, non-hydrogenated margarine or mayonnaise
2 tsp (10 mL) low-fat mayonnaise, cream cheese or peanut butter
1-2 tbsp (15-25 mL) low-fat salad dressing
6 olives

* Serving sizes are per Canada's Food Guide to Healthy Eating. Check U.S. Food Guide Pyramid for corresponding serving sizes. This eating plan provides approximately 1500 calories per day.

# Healthy Eating Plan III*

7 Grain Products
3 Vegetables (or more) and 4 Fruit
3 Milk Products

3 Meat and Alternatives
5-6 Fats and Oils (Other Foods)

**Breakfast:**

| | |
|---|---|
| 2 Grain | 2 slices toast or 2 oz (50g) cold unsweetened cereal or 1½ cup (375 mL) hot cereal |
| 1 Fruit | one medium orange or ½ cup (125 mL) berries |
| 1 Milk | 1 cup (250 mL) skim milk or ¾ cup fat-free yogurt |

**Lunch:**

| | |
|---|---|
| 2 Grain | 2 slices bread or 2 oz (50g) bagel or roll |
| 1 Vegetable | 1 cup (250 mL) salad or vegetable soup |
| 1 Meat | 2-3 oz (50-100 g) turkey slices or ½ cup (125 mL) water-packed tuna |
| 2 Fat | 2 tsp (10 mL) low-fat mayo + 2 tbsp (25 mL) low-fat salad dressing or 2 tsp (10 mL) oil |

**Snack:**

| | |
|---|---|
| 1 Grain | 4 melba toast |
| 1 Fruit | ½ cup (125 mL) mixed fruit |
| 1 Milk | ¾ cup (175 mL) fat-free yogurt |

**Dinner:**

| | |
|---|---|
| 2 Grain | 1 cup (250 mL) rice or pasta or 2 slices bread |
| 2 Vegetable | ½ cup (125 mL) peas and ½ cup (125 mL) cooked broccoli |
| 1 Fruit | 1 baked apple |
| 2 Meat | 6 oz (175 g) lean poultry, meat or fish or 1½ cup (375 mL) beans |
| 3-4 Fat | 3-4 tsp (15-20 mL) oil |

**Snack:**

| | |
|---|---|
| 1 Fruit | medium banana |
| 1 Milk | 1 cup (250 mL) lite hot chocolate |

**Fats and Oils Choices (Other Foods):**
1 tsp (5 mL) oil, non-hydrogenated margarine or mayonnaise
2 tsp (10 mL) low-fat mayonnaise, cream cheese or peanut butter
1-2 tbsp (15-25 mL) low-fat salad dressing
6 olives

* Serving sizes are per Canada's Food Guide to Healthy Eating. Check U.S. Food Guide Pyramid for corresponding serving sizes. This eating plan provides approximately 1800 calories per day.

## The Lighten Up Way

*We remove some of the fat, make lighter choices and keep portion sizes in line with the food guides recommended serving sizes.*

Another way to create your own healthy eating plan is to lighten up the way you're eating now. You can trim your current intake down to size by doing a little fine-tuning. I do this with my clients all the time. We remove some of the fat, make lighter choices and keep portion sizes in line with the food guide's recommended serving sizes.

You can do this for yourself too. Start by taking a look at your usual breakfast. It might be a toasted bagel spread with cream cheese, and a cup of coffee with cream and sugar. You can lighten up by switching the bagel to one slice of whole wheat toast and substituting fruit spread for the cream cheese. Balance it with a serving of fruit and fat-free yogurt, and have your coffee with a splash of milk instead of cream. You'll be satisfied until lunch, you're getting more food than before and you've cut your intake of fat and calories. For variety, how about a serving of whole grain hot or cold cereal with berries and skim milk?

Let's see how much fat and how many calories you can save without going on any diet disasters, just by lightening up what you're eating now.

# What You're Eating Now

| Meal | Choose Instead | Save (approx) Fat | Calories |
|------|----------------|-----|----------|
| **Breakfast** | | | |
| 1 bagel | 1 slice wheat toast, fruit spread | 0 | 107 |
| 2 tbsp (25 mL) cream cheese | ¾ cup (175 mL) fat-free yogurt | 10 | 30 |
| 1 cup (250 mL) orange juice | 1 orange | 0 | 36 |
| coffee with cream | coffee with skim milk | 5 | 44 |
| **Lunch** | | | |
| tuna with mayo | turkey with mustard | 13 | 138 |
| on a bagel | on rye bread | 0 | 29 |
| 1 oz (30 g) potato chips | salad, 1 tsp (15 mL) oil, vinegar | 5 | 85 |
| donut | 1 cup fruit salad | 10 | 74 |
| 12 oz (355 mL) soft drink | 1 cup (250 mL) tomato juice | 0 | 100 |
| **Snack** | | | |
| 2 chocolate chip cookies | 4 melba toast with fruit spread | 4 | 17 |
| 1 cup (250 mL) 2% milk | 1 cup (250 mL) skim milk | 4 | 30 |
| **Dinner** | | | |
| 1 baked potato | 1 baked potato | 0 | 0 |
| 1 tbsp (15 mL) sour cream | 1 tbsp (15 mL) salsa | 5 | 47 |
| 1 cup (250 mL) broccoli | 1 cup (250 mL) broccoli | 0 | 0 |
| 1 tbsp (15 mL) butter | 1 tsp (5 mL) non-hydrogenated margarine | 7 | 65 |
| 6 oz (175 g) steak, untrimmed | 3 oz (100g) steak, trimmed | 31 | 341 |
| apple pie | baked apple | 12 | 200 |

**Total Saved   106 g fat 1343 cal.**

Seeing is believing! By making lighter food choices and trimming portion sizes, over a hundred grams of fat and more than one thousand calories have been eliminated. Remember, we said that you need to pare down your intake by 3500 calories to reduce your body weight by one pound. This means that if you lighten up by 500 calories each day while still eating in a healthy way, you'll be trimming off one pound (0.5 kg) per week. When you do this consistently, your healthy weight goal will become a reality in no time. Add in that activity we talked about earlier, and you'll reach and maintain your goal with ease.

## Vitality

A wonderful message on Canada's Food Guide is expressed in the very last line: "Enjoy eating well, being active and feeling good about yourself. That's vitality."

*Feeling good about yourself means believing in yourself and treating yourself well.*

I love this message because to me, that's what seeing the light is all about too—eating in a lighter, healthier way and being active by moving your body and having fun. Feeling good about yourself means believing in yourself and treating yourself well. All these elements work together to help you achieve your healthy eating, weight and lifestyle goals, once and for all.

Years ago, when I embarked on my journey to achieve a healthier lifestyle, I started keeping an assortment of health and nutrition books, magazines and cookbooks on my night table in my bedroom. They were good company. They motivated and inspired me to eat in a healthy way, feel good about myself and enjoy what I was doing.

Whenever I'd feel the urge to snack, instead of raiding the cookie jar I would go up to my bedroom and read my books. I'd feed my mind, heart and soul. Later when I became a dietitian, I pledged that I would write the book I wish I'd had on my night table all those years.

Well, dear friend, I've finally written that book. It's for you, to show you how to make the changes in your life that will lead to a lighter, healthier, happier you. I hope you will keep it by your side to read and reread, to inspire, educate and motivate you to keep going, even when things may not be moving along as well as you might want. And it's for me too, for now I've fulfilled the promise that I made to us all.

This book is your companion on your journey to living life in a healthy way. Keep it by your side and your goals will always be within your reach. Every day, open it and read a few pages. Review your snack attack strategy, make a new recipe or plan a non-food reward. I know you'll stay excited about healthy eating and the good things that you're doing for yourself. You can and will succeed as long as you believe in yourself and keep "seeing the light".

> *This book is your companion on your journey to living life in a healthy way. Keep it by your side and your goals will always be within your reach.*

# PART 2

# Recipes for Success

*T*HE "RECIPES FOR SUCCESS" will show you how to cook the foods you love to eat in a lighter and healthier way. You'll also see that you can enjoy many of your own favorite recipes just by cutting back on much of the fat.

You may be wondering where my light and easy recipes came from. The truth is, all I did was lighten up the way I used to cook. I took my favorite recipes and slashed the fat and calories, but not the taste. No way! I was never going to deprive myself again. I know now that deprivation only leads to the misery of binge eating. Melba toast and celery sticks are okay, but it's no way to live.

So, on a Sunday morning, you can usually find me at the supermarket. After the hectic pace of a work week, I enjoy a leisurely stroll through the supermarket aisles to shop and check out what's new in the food world. I'm probably thinking about a request or two from my clients for an easy low-fat recipe, maybe a soup, a fish dish or a baked fruit dessert.

When I come home from shopping, inspired by all the fresh and wonderful foods I've seen, I start cooking. Today, it was a California vegetable soup and an apple raisin crisp. I use simple ingredients because I believe in the "KISS" formula of cuisine. No, not the rock group. The "Keep It Simple, Sweetie" method.

*Keeping fat and calories low lets my clients and me achieve and maintain our healthy weight goals.*

I use little or no added fat because I believe food doesn't need a lot of fat to taste good. Just wait until you try some of these recipes. You'll see what I mean. Keeping fat and calories low lets my clients and me achieve and maintain our healthy weight goals. Don't forget, I may be the head of the healthy eating class, but I'm still a member.

The first recipe I created was Speedy Vegetarian Chili. Early on in my practice, I was counselling a client on the cholesterol-lowering benefits of consuming the soluble fiber found in dried beans, peas and lentils. He said that he'd like to give those legumes a try, but how was he supposed to eat them. He didn't relish the idea of living on endless tins of baked beans in tomato sauce.

I wasn't sure what to tell him since I myself had never cooked a bean dish in my life. So I decided that I would experiment with vegetarian chili, a one pot meal that seemed like something anyone could make, even me, inexperienced as I was in bean cuisine.

I had several cans of chickpeas and kidney beans in my pantry that I had planned to do something with someday when I got around to it. Well, someday had finally come. The great chili cookoff was about to begin.

First, I chopped a small onion and cooked it until it was fragrant in a teaspoon or two of canola oil. Next, I added sliced celery and carrots and continued to cook the vegetables until they were softened. (These days, I just soften the onion and veggies in a little bit of water.) So far, so good, I figured. I drained a can of chickpeas, kidney beans, and mushrooms that I found in my pantry and dumped them into the pot. Next, in with some canned tomatoes, a splash of tomato juice, some seasonings and parsley. I let my chili simmer for about twenty minutes. It smelled great, but how would it taste? I dipped my spoon into the simmering mixture, took a mouthful, closed my eyes and swallowed.

Ay Chihuahua! It was delicious. Nobody was more surprised than I was. I served it to my family, the toughest food critics in the world, I might add. When they kept eating and started asking for seconds, I knew I had a winner.

I made copies of the recipe, gave one to my client and the rest to my other clients and members of The Fitness Institute. This was the first of many. Before long, I had a collection of terrific recipes that everyone was enjoying and sharing with family and friends. Nothing could be finer than

*Before long, I had a collection of terrific recipes that everyone was enjoying and sharing with family and friends.*

hearing from a client that his or her family or guests loved one of my recipes and never guessed that it was good for them too.

The recipes have become an important part of my nutrition practice. As my clients keep busy shopping for, preparing and enjoying the healthy recipes, they stay focused on what they can eat, instead of feeling deprived and unhappy about all the foods they shouldn't be eating. They feel good about themselves, they're awakening their tastebuds to the incredible taste of lighter food and they're replacing guilt and deprivation with satisfaction and enjoyment. They're seeing the light just by making some simple recipes. And so will you.

## CHAPTER 11

# Breakfast for Champions

$\mathcal{E}$ATING BREAKFAST starts your day off right. If you're not hungry for breakfast, maybe too much evening snacking is to blame. When you start eating in a lighter way, you should feel comfortably hungry in the morning, ready to enjoy your first meal of the day.

After a night-time fast, eating a balanced breakfast boosts low blood sugar and energizes your morning. You may think that skipping breakfast is an easy way to save three hundred calories or more. On the contrary. Studies show that people who skip breakfast tend to more than make up for the missed calories later in the day, but not the nutrients. It's pretty hard to avoid the siren's call of that mid-morning donut and coffee on an empty stomach. Eating breakfast will help curb cravings and keep you satisfied until lunch.

Many clients report that they don't like eating breakfast because it makes them feel hungrier throughout the day. That's probably true, but it's not a bad thing. They're probably hungry because their bodies are burning calories instead of holding onto them.

Conserving calories is something your body does when you go for long periods of time without eating. Your body

*After a night-time fast, eating a balanced breakfast boosts low blood sugar and energizes your morning.*

doesn't know the difference between your decision to skip breakfast and you being stranded on a desert island with nothing to eat. It assumes you're going into starvation mode and hangs on to every calorie as long as it can, which is exactly what you don't want. Eating helps burn calories. But remember, we're talking about healthy eating.

Your breakfast doesn't have to be fancy or take a long time to eat. It can be as simple as a cup of hot or cold cereal, skim milk and a fruit; or a slice of toast, small container of fat-free yogurt and a banana; or a toasted English muffin, one-minute microwave egg whites and sliced tomato. A great portable breakfast is a home-made low-fat muffin, an orange and a carton of skim milk.

> *A great portable breakfast is a home-made low-fat muffin, an orange and a carton of skim milk.*

On the weekend when you have more time, treat yourself to a brunch of Berry Good French Toast. Or pop half a bagel in the toaster and give it a light coating of Creamy Dreamy Yogurt Cheese. Tuck into a bowl of Hawaiian Fruit Salad. Put on a pot of coffee, turn on some classical music and curl up with the weekend paper. Take your time and pamper yourself. You deserve it.

## Breakfast Basics

1. A balanced breakfast includes at least three food groups: a grain product like bread or cereal, a vegetable or fruit, and a source of protein which can be a milk product or a meat alternative like low-fat cheese, fish or egg whites.

2. Keep breakfast low in fat. Choose whole grain breads and cereals with no more than 1 gram fat per serving, and skim or 1% milk, cottage cheese or yogurt. Enjoy toast with fruit spread instead of butter or margarine. Avoid granola-type cereals, croissants and regular muffins which can be loaded with fat and calories.

3. Whenever possible eat a fruit instead of drinking fruit juice to get the benefit of the fiber in the whole fruit. If a whole fruit is not available or practical, fruit juice will do. But generally, it's better to eat your fruit and drink water when you're thirsty.

4. Keep low-fat muffins in the freezer to keep them fresher longer. They tend to get stale quickly because of their lower fat content. Thaw and warm your muffin in the microwave or toaster-oven before eating to give it that "just baked" taste we all love. Keeping the muffins frozen will also remove the temptation to eat more than just one. No "multiple" muffins for us.

5. If you're on the road or at a breakfast meeting, good restaurant choices include hot or cold cereal with skim milk, toasted English muffin or bagel with jam, pancakes with a bit of syrup, egg white omelette, whole grain toast, low-fat cottage cheese or yogurt and fresh fruit. Avoid high fat/high calorie items like regular fried eggs and omelettes, breakfast meats and baked goods.

*Keeping the muffins frozen will also remove the temptation to eat more than just one. No "multiple" muffins for us.*

# Breakfast Recipes

# Apple Butter Bran Muffins

The secret ingredient in these high fiber, low-fat muffins is apple butter, which isn't butter at all. It's just spreadable apples.

| | | |
|---|---|---|
| 2 tbsp | canola oil | 25 mL |
| 4 | egg whites or ½ cup/125 mL egg whites in a carton | 4 |
| 1 tsp | vanilla | 5 mL |
| ½ cup | orange juice | 125 mL |
| 3 tbsp | apple butter | 45 mL |
| ½ cup | skim milk | 125 mL |
| 1½ cups | whole wheat flour | 375 mL |
| 2 cups | bran cereal (with 10 grams fiber per serving) | 500 mL |
| ¼ cup | sugar | 50 mL |
| 1 tsp | baking soda | 5 mL |
| 2 tsp | baking powder | 10 mL |
| ½ tsp | cinnamon | 2 mL |
| ½ cup | raisins | 125 mL |

**The Lowdown**
(per muffin)

| | |
|---|---|
| calories | 155 |
| fat | 3 g |
| carbohydrate | 32 g |
| protein | 5 g |

**Highlight**

Each muffin provides 6 grams fiber.

1. Combine wet ingredients in a bowl.
2. In a larger bowl combine dry ingredients.
3. Pour wet ingredients over dry ingredients and stir to combine. Stir in raisins
4. Spoon into paper-lined or non-stick muffin tins.
5. Bake in a 375°F/190°C oven for 15 to 18 minutes.

Makes 12 muffins.

# Going Bananas Muffins

This is a basic muffin recipe that offers lots of yummy options. You can substitute dried cranberries, currants or raisins for the chocolate chips. For added kid-appeal, top these muffins with colored sprinkles, a tip I got from my daughter Michelle, who is a pre-school teacher. Your kids will want to help you make and eat these muffins too.

| | | |
|---|---|---|
| 2 tbsp | soft margarine | 25 mL |
| 1/3 cup | white sugar | 75 mL |
| 4 | egg whites or 1/2 cup/125 mL egg whites in a carton, lightly beaten | 4 |
| 1 tsp | vanilla | 5 mL |
| 3 | ripe bananas, mashed | 3 |
| 1/2 cup | skim milk | 125 mL |
| 1 cup each | whole wheat and all-purpose flour | 250 mL each |
| 1 tsp | baking soda | 5 mL |
| 2 tsp | baking powder | 10 mL |
| 1/2 cup | chocolate chips | 125 mL |

1. In a large bowl, cream together margarine and sugar. Stir in egg whites, vanilla, mashed bananas and skim milk.
2. In a separate bowl combine flour, baking soda and baking powder.
3. Stir dry ingredients into wet ingredients until well combined and not lumpy. Stir in chocolate chips.
4. Spoon into paper-lined or non-stick muffin tins.
5. Bake in a 375°F/190°C oven for about 20 to 25 minutes until golden brown.

Makes 12 muffins.

# No Loafin' Zucchini Loaf

This recipe is a lightened up version of a family favorite that was loaded with fat and calories. The applesauce, raisins and high water content in the zucchini make this loaf moist and tender.

| | The Lowdown (per slice) | |
|---|---|---|
| calories | | 176 |
| fat | | 3 g |
| carbohydrate | | 34 g |
| protein | | 5 g |

| | | |
|---|---|---|
| 2 tbsp | canola oil | 25 mL |
| ¾ cup | unsweetened applesauce | 175 mL |
| 4 | egg whites or ½ cup/125 mL egg whites in a carton, lightly beaten | 4 |
| ⅓ cup | sugar | 75 mL |
| 1 tsp | vanilla | 5 mL |
| 1 cup | raw zucchini, grated | 250 mL |
| 1 cup each | whole wheat and all-purpose flour | 250 mL each |
| 1 tsp | baking soda | 5 mL |
| 1 tsp | baking powder | 5 mL |
| 1 tsp | cinnamon | 5 mL |
| ¼ tsp | salt | 1 mL |
| ½ cup | raisins | 125 mL |
| | cooking spray | |

1. In a large mixing bowl, combine oil, applesauce, egg whites, sugar and vanilla. Blend well. Stir in zucchini.
2. Combine flour, baking soda, baking powder, cinnamon and salt. Add to liquid ingredients and stir until not lumpy.
3. Stir in raisins. Pour mixture into a loaf pan sprayed with cooking spray.
4. Bake in a 325°F/160°C oven for 1 hour.

Makes 1 loaf, 10 slices.

# Egg White Omelette

**The Lowdown**
(per omelette)

| | |
|---|---|
| calories | 66 |
| fat | 1 g |
| carbohydrate | 3 g |
| protein | 12 g |

**Highlight**

For a cheese omelette, sprinkle with part-skim Mozzarella cheese before folding. To go Mexican top with 2 tbsp/25 mL salsa.

Have you ever tried making an egg white omelette and ended up with a frisbee on a plate? If you have, you're not the only one. The trick to turning out perfect egg whites is "low and slow". Cook on medium to low heat and take your time. Without the fat that's found in the yolk, your gentle egg whites won't take the rigors of cooking too quickly on high heat. And if you can't get used to the white color, a pinch of turmeric will turn your egg whites golden.

| 4 | egg whites or | 4 |
|---|---|---|
| | ½ cup/125 mL egg whites in a carton | |
| | pinch turmeric (optional) | |
| | pepper, fresh herbs (to taste) | |
| | cooking spray | |
| | tomato or orange slice (optional) | |

1. Whisk egg whites until frothy.
2. Heat an 8-inch/20 cm non-stick pan sprayed with cooking spray.
3. Pour egg whites into pan and cook on medium heat until egg whites start to set.
4. Sprinkle pepper and herbs over egg whites.
5. Fold over or turn omelette and cook until no longer translucent.
6. Serve garnished with a slice of orange or tomato.

Makes 1 omelette.

# Light and Easy Frittata

Enjoy this light and easy frittata for brunch, teamed with half a toasted bagel and sliced tomatoes. For dinner add a salad, small potato and fruit for dessert.

| 4 | egg whites or | 4 |
| | ½ cup/125 mL egg whites in a carton | |
| ½ cup | fresh or frozen mixed vegetables | 125 mL |
| | (broccoli, carrots, mushrooms, | |
| | onion, peppers) | |
| | cooking spray | |
| | fresh or dried herbs (to taste) | |
| | salt, pepper (to taste) | |

**The Lowdown**
(per frittata)

| | |
|---|---|
| calories | 85 |
| fat | 1 g |
| carbohydrate | 7 g |
| protein | 13 g |

1. Soften vegetables in microwave or steam for 1-2 minutes. Pour off water.
2. Beat egg whites. Combine with softened vegetables, herbs, salt and pepper, to taste.
3. Pour mixture into a small heated pan sprayed with cooking spray.
4. Cook on medium to low heat until frittata is set.
5. Carefully turn frittata and cook until frittata is golden brown.

Makes 1 frittata.

# Berry Good French Toast

**The Lowdown**
**(per serving)**

| | |
|---|---:|
| calories | 125 |
| fat | 2 g |
| carbohydrate | 18 g |
| protein | 9 g |

What a fabulous combo—golden brown French toast and tart-sweet berries! Spoil yourself by buying the most luscious berries you can find, even in winter.

| | | |
|---|---|---|
| 8 | egg whites or | 8 |
| | 1 cup/250 mL egg whites in a carton | |
| ¼ cup | skim milk | 50 mL |
| 4 | slices bread, preferably whole wheat | 4 |
| ½ tsp | vanilla | 2 mL |
| ¼ tsp | cinnamon | 1 mL |
| | cooking spray | |
| 1 cup | fresh berries (blueberries, | 250 mL |
| | sliced strawberries, raspberries) | |
| | icing sugar (optional) | |
| | maple syrup (optional) | |
| | fresh mint (optional) | |

1. Whisk egg whites with skim milk, vanilla and cinnamon.
2. Pour egg white mixture into a large flat dish. Dip each bread slice in egg white mixture and turn to coat both sides.
3. Heat a large non-stick pan sprayed with cooking spray.
4. On medium heat brown the bread slices. Turn to cook both sides.
5. To serve, place 1 slice French toast on a plate. Top with ¼ cup/50 mL fresh berries. Dust with icing sugar and a drizzle of maple syrup, if desired. Garnish with a sprig of fresh mint.

Makes 4 servings.

# Hawaiian Fruit Salad

Don't be surprised if you feel like doing the Hula dance when you taste this exotic fruit salad. The orange juice will keep the fruit fresh in the refrigerator for 3-5 days, or until it disappears, whichever comes first.

| | | |
|---|---|---|
| 1 | cantaloupe, peeled, seeded and cubed | 1 |
| 1 | golden pineapple, peeled, cored and cut in chunks | 1 |
| 2 cups | strawberries, washed, hulled and sliced | 500 mL |
| 3 | kiwi, peeled and sliced | 3 |
| ¾ cup | orange juice | 175 mL |

1. Arrange fresh fruit in a large bowl. Pour over orange juice.
2. Cover bowl with plastic wrap and refrigerate.

Makes 16 servings, ½ cup each.

**The Lowdown**
**(per ½ cup/125 mL)**

| | |
|---|---|
| calories | 50 |
| fat | 0 g |
| carbohydrate | 12 g |
| protein | 1 g |

**The Lowdown**

For an afternoon snack, top with fat-free yogurt and a sprinkle of wheat germ.

# What's the Story, Morning Glory?

| **The Lowdown** (per serving) | |
| --- | --- |
| calories | 221 |
| fat | 1 g |
| carbohydrate | 41 g |
| protein | 13 g |

If you're lactose intolerant like I am, this combo with low-lactose yogurt starts your day with an excellent boost of calcium. It's well-balanced because it contains three of the four food groups, it's low in fat and tastes delicious.

| ½ cup | Hawaiian Fruit Salad | 125 mL |
| ¾ cup | plain fat-free yogurt | 175 mL |
| 1 | packet sweetener (optional) | 1 |
| 1 slice | whole grain toast | 1 slice |
| 2 tsp | fruit spread | 10 mL |

1. Place fruit in a cereal bowl. Top with yogurt and sweetener, if using.
2. To complete your breakfast, add one slice whole grain toast topped with fruit spread and a hot beverage.

Makes 1 serving.

# Oh You Smoothie

Turn this smoothie into an amazing fat-free milk shake by adding a few ice cubes and substituting ½ cup fresh or frozen strawberries for the banana.

| | | |
|---|---|---|
| ¾ cup | plain fat-free yogurt | 175 mL |
| ½ cup | orange juice | 125 mL |
| ½ | ripe banana | ½ |
| | sweetener (optional) | |

1. Whirl ingredients together in a blender or food processor until fruit is puréed. Pour into a tall glass and enjoy.

Makes 1 smoothie.

**The Lowdown**
(per smoothie)

| | |
|---|---|
| calories | 199 |
| fat | 0 g |
| carbohydrate | 40 g |
| protein | 11 g |

# Dreamy Creamy Yogurt Cheese

This is the light stuff, a delicious substitute for that higher-fat spread. Spice it up if you wish with some fresh dill or chives and lots of fresh ground pepper. Or go sweet with some crushed pineapple. Spread plain yogurt cheese on half a toasted bagel and top with a slice of lox, tomato, onion and capers. A dream come true!

| | | |
|---|---|---|
| 2 cups | plain fat-free yogurt with no added gels or thickeners | 500 mL |

1. Line a strainer with cheesecloth, coffee filter or 2 paper towels, and place over a bowl.
2. Place yogurt in the strainer and cover with plastic wrap.
3. Place in refrigerator overnight.
4. Discard drained liquid and spoon yogurt cheese into a clean bowl.
5. Cover and refrigerate for up to one week.

Makes 1 cup yogurt cheese.

**The Lowdown**
(per 1 tbsp /15 mL)

| | |
|---|---|
| calories | 7 |
| fat | 0 g |
| carbohydrate | 1 g |
| protein | 1 g |

# One-Minute "Poached" Egg Whites on Toast

## The Lowdown
(per serving)

| | |
|---|---|
| calories | 98 |
| fat | 1 g |
| carbohydrate | 14 g |
| protein | 9 g |

These egg whites cook in one minute in the microwave, probably faster than it takes to toast the bread. Great for breakfast with a dab of ketchup or a slice of tomato, for lunch with soup or salad, or for a pre-party snack to help curb a ravenous appetite and help you avoid high-fat finger food.

| | | |
|---|---|---|
| 2 | egg whites or ¼ cup/50 mL egg whites in a carton | 2 |
| 1 | slice whole wheat bread | 1 |
| | pepper, onion flakes, herbs (optional) | |

1. In a small glass bowl, lightly beat egg whites. Add seasonings, if desired.
2. Cover and microwave on High for 1 minute, or until egg whites are no long translucent.
3. Toast 1 slice of whole wheat bread.
4. Place cooked egg whites on toast.

Makes 1 serving.

# Grown-Up Peanut Butter and Banana on Toast

Just in case I've given you the impression that peanut butter is off limits, I thought I would include one of my favorite combos for you to try. Even though peanut butter is high in fat and calories, it's a nutrient-dense food, which means it packs a lot of nutrition into a small portion. Just remember to count it as a fat choice and enjoy.

| 1 slice | whole wheat bread | 1 slice |
| 2 tsp | natural peanut butter | 10 mL |
| ½ | banana, sliced in rounds | ½ |

1. Toast 1 slice whole wheat bread.
2. Spread toast thinly with peanut butter.
3. Top with banana slices.

Makes 1 serving.

**The Lowdown**
(per serving)

| | |
|---|---|
| calories | 177 |
| fat | 6 g |
| carbohydrate | 27 g |
| protein | 6 g |

**Highlight**

To lighten up on the fat and calories, you can pour off some of the oil from the top of the natural peanut butter. Natural peanut butter is recommended because it is not hydrogenated and therefore contains no "trans" fat.

CHAPTER 12

# Salad Days

S ALAD HAS COME A LONG WAY from the standard iceberg lettuce, watery tomato and limp cucumber combo of the past. New and interesting greens, lower fat dressings and flavored vinegars make salad a satisfying part of a meal instead of the dieter's ration of rabbit food. With bagged pre-washed lettuce and salad ingredients available in most supermarkets, there's almost no excuse for going a day without salad.

Including a salad with your meal will take the edge off your hunger. It's a sure-fire way to lighten up your intake and your waistline. But be careful with the dressing. Case in point: that meal-size Caesar you order as a virtuous lunch can pack hundreds of calories and a day's worth of fat. So when ordering your salad in a restaurant, be sure to ask for a wedge of lemon, vinegar or vinaigrette dressing on the side.

At home, dress your salads with balsamic, raspberry, tarragon, rice or wine vinegar. These can be enjoyed alone or with a tiny bit of olive or canola oil. The oil will help the dressing cling to the leaves.

When I created my first low-fat vinaigrette, I added a little sweetener to cut the tartness of the vinegar. You can do the same or add a pinch of sugar instead, if you wish. I also

*With bagged pre-washed lettuce and salad ingredients available in most supermarkets, there's almost no excuse for going a day without salad.*

*Want a creamy dressing? You'd be amazed what a spoonful of fat-free yogurt or Dijon mustard can do.*

added some water. If adding water to salad dressing sounds strange to you, check out the ingredients on the label of a low-fat dressing in your refrigerator. You'll see that one of the first ingredients is water. Want a creamy dressing? You'd be amazed what a spoonful of fat-free yogurt or Dijon mustard can do.

Salad can also double as a complete meal. Just add a source of protein like chickpeas, water-packed tuna, grated low-fat feta cheese, sliced grilled chicken, soy veggie "turkey", or chopped hard-boiled egg or egg whites. Team your salad with a slice of whole grain bread or a roll and a piece of fruit for dessert. And of course, dress your salad with one of my delicious low-fat dressings. Voila! Your salad has just turned into a light and easy lunch or supper. Your waistline will thank you.

## Salad Solutions

1. Bagged pre-washed lettuce and salad ingredients may cost a little more, but as I've mentioned before, it's worth it if you actually eat the greens instead of having to throw them out because you haven't had time to wash and chop.

2. Keep a bowl of undressed salad in the refrigerator. This way your salad will be ready to wrap and tuck into a brown bag to go, to team with a sandwich for lunch or to enjoy as an appetizer before dinner without a lot of last-minute fuss and bother.

3. Be adventurous with your salad vegetables. Try a rainbow of peppers in red, yellow and orange instead of your standard green. English cucumbers, cherry tomatoes, spring onions, water chestnuts, baby corn, shredded carrots, purple cabbage, hearts of palm, bean and

pea sprouts, mushrooms, celery, broccoli florets and asparagus spears, toss them in.

4. For maximum nutrition choose deep-colored green, orange and red vegetables.

5. Seasoned rice vinegar makes a delicious fat-free salad dressing on its own. The touch of salt and sugar adds a lot of flavor and not many calories.

6. Be careful with bottled fat-free or low-fat salad dressings. Fat-free doesn't mean calorie-free, so pour with a light hand. The taste of some fat-free dressings can be disappointing. Use them for convenience if you find one that you enjoy. Or make one you'll really love using the recipes in this chapter.

*Seasoned rice vinegar makes a delicious fat-free salad dressing on its own. The touch of salt and sugar adds a lot of flavor and not many calories.*

# Salad Recipes

# Mexicali Black Bean and Corn Salad

This fiber-rich salad travels south of the border for its vibrant taste and fabulous colors.

| | | |
|---|---|---|
| 1 | 19 oz / 540 mL can black beans, drained and rinsed | 1 |
| 1½ cups | cooked corn niblets | 375 mL |
| ½ each | red and green pepper, seeded and diced | ½ each |
| 2 oz | red onion, diced | 50 g |
| 1 | tomato, diced | 1 |

**Dressing:**

| | | |
|---|---|---|
| 1 tbsp | canola oil | 15 mL |
| 1 tbsp | lime juice | 15 mL |
| ¼ cup | red wine vinegar | 50 mL |
| ½ tsp | salt (or to taste) | 2 mL |
| | fresh ground pepper | |
| ½ tsp | garlic powder | 2 mL |
| ½ tsp | dried cilantro | 2 mL |
| 1 | packet sweetener or 2 tsp/10 mL sugar | 1 |

1. In a bowl, combine black beans, corn niblets, diced peppers, onion and tomato.
2. In a separate bowl, combine dressing ingredients. Pour over black bean mixture and stir gently to combine.
3. Cover bowl and refrigerate for 2 hours or overnight.

Makes 8 servings.

**The Lowdown**
(per serving)

| | |
|---|---|
| calories | 109 |
| fat | 2 g |
| carbohydrate | 19 g |
| protein | 5 g |

**Highlight**

Serve cold as a main dish on a bed of greens, or as a salsa with grilled fish or chicken.

# Oo La La! Salad Niçoise

This main-course salad is popular in the south of France. The oil-rich dressing, olives and hard-cooked eggs "can can" add lots of fat and calories. Try this svelte version to kick up your tastebuds.

| | The Lowdown (per serving) | |
| --- | --- | --- |
| calories | | 245 |
| fat | | 8 g |
| carbohydrate | | 25 g |
| protein | | 21 g |

| | | |
| --- | --- | --- |
| 4 cups | salad greens, washed, dried and torn in pieces | 1 L |
| 2 | 6 oz/170 g cans solid water-packed tuna, drained | 2 |
| ½ lb | green beans, blanched | 250 g |
| 4 | small red potatoes, cooked, cut in quarters | 4 |
| 2 | tomatoes, cut in wedges | 2 |
| 1 | hard-boiled egg, cut in quarters | 1 |
| 8 | black olives | 8 |
| 4 | anchovies (optional) | 4 |

**Dressing:**

| | | |
| --- | --- | --- |
| 1 tbsp | canola oil | 15 mL |
| 2 tbsp | water | 25 mL |
| ¼ cup | red wine vinegar | 50 mL |
| 2 tsp | sugar or equivalent sweetener | 10 mL |
| ½ tsp | garlic powder | 2 mL |
| ½ tsp | dried tarragon | 2 mL |
| ½ tsp | dried thyme | 2 mL |
| 2 tbsp | red onion, minced | 25 mL |
| ½ tsp | salt (or to taste) | 2 mL |
| | ground black pepper (to taste) | |

1. Place salad greens in a large salad bowl. In center of greens, arrange tuna in chunks.
2. In pinwheel fashion, arrange green beans, potato, egg quarters and tomato wedges. Garnish with black olives and drained, rinsed anchovies, if using.
3. In a small bowl, whisk together salad dressing ingredients.
4. Just before serving, drizzle dressing over salad or serve dressing on the side.

Makes 4 servings.

# *Jerusalem Salad*

In the Middle East, this salad is served for breakfast with bread and yogurt, for lunch with hummus and pita, and for dinner with grilled chicken or fish. You can enjoy this salad at home and let your tastebuds do the travelling.

| ½ | English cucumber, diced | ½ |
|---|---|---|
| 1 | large tomato, diced | 1 |
| 2 tbsp | parsley, chopped | 25 mL |
| 1 tbsp | olive oil | 15 mL |
| | juice of ½ a lemon | |
| | salt (to taste) | |
| | ground black pepper (to taste) | |

1. Combine vegetables and parsley in a bowl.
2. Add olive oil, lemon juice, salt and pepper to taste. Stir and chill before serving.

Makes 6 servings.

**The Lowdown**
(per serving)

| | |
|---|---|
| calories | 31 |
| fat | 2 g |
| carbohydrate | 2 g |
| protein | 1 g |

**Highlight**

Use 2 or 3 small plum tomatoes instead of 1 large tomato. Plum tomatoes have less juice and seeds which makes them easier to dice. Or you can gently squeeze out the juice and seeds from your tomato before dicing.

# Healthy Hummus

**The Lowdown**
**(per 1 tbsp / 15 mL)**

| | |
|---|---|
| calories | 15 |
| fat | 0 g |
| carbohydrate | 3 g |
| protein | 1 g |

You can make this hummus any time, as long as you have a can of chickpeas in your pantry. A client told me she served this recipe to a guest from the Middle East and he loved it. To me, that's a standing ovation.

| | | |
|---|---|---|
| 1 | 19 oz/540 mL can chickpeas, drained (reserve ¼ cup liquid) | 1 |
| 2 tbsp | ultra-light or fat-free mayonnaise | 25 mL |
| 1 tsp | natural peanut butter or tahini | 5 mL |
| | juice of ½ a lemon | |
| ½ tsp each | garlic powder, black pepper, ground cumin (or to taste) | 2 mL each |

1. Place ingredients in bowl of food processor. Purée until well blended and fairly smooth, adding reserved liquid from chickpeas to obtain desired consistency. Pour mixture into a bowl, cover and refrigerate until serving time.
2. Serve as a dip or spread with pita bread or raw vegetables.

Makes 2 cups/500 mL hummus.

# Mandarin Salad

Intensely-flavored sesame oil packs a huge amount of taste into a few drops. The little bit of extra fat and calories are worth it.

| | | |
|---|---|---|
| 4 cups | mixed greens, rinsed and dried | 1 L |
| ½ lb | white mushrooms, washed and sliced | 250 g |
| ¼ lb | bean sprouts, rinsed | 125 g |
| ½ | red pepper, washed and cut in thin strips | ½ |
| ½ | red onion, thinly sliced | ½ |
| 1 cup | sliced water chestnuts, | 250 mL |
| 1 | 14 oz / 398 mL can baby corn, drained and rinsed | 1 |
| 1 | 10 oz / 284 mL can mandarin orange segments, drained | 1 |

**Dressing:**

| | | |
|---|---|---|
| 1 tbsp | sesame oil | 15 mL |
| 2 tbsp | water | 25 mL |
| 2 tbsp | low-sodium soy sauce | 25 mL |
| ¼ cup | seasoned rice vinegar | 50 mL |
| 1 | clove garlic, minced | 1 |
| ½ tsp | black pepper | 2 mL |

1. In a large bowl combine salad ingredients.
2. In a small bowl whisk together dressing.
3. Just before serving, toss salad with dressing or serve dressing on the side.

Makes 4 servings.

**The Lowdown**
(per serving)

| | |
|---|---|
| calories | 167 |
| fat | 4 g |
| carbohydrate | 28 g |
| protein | 6 g |

# Santorini Salad

**The Lowdown**
(per serving)

| | |
|---|---|
| calories | 157 |
| fat | 11 g |
| carbohydrate | 11 g |
| protein | 6 g |

Named for one of the most beautiful of the Hellenic islands, this salad is a new spin on a Greek classic.

| | | |
|---|---|---|
| 4 cups | lettuce leaves, rinsed, dried and torn in pieces | 1 L |
| ½ | cucumber, cut in chunks | ½ |
| ½ each | red and green pepper, cut in chunks | ½ each |
| 2 | tomatoes, cut in wedges | 2 |
| 4 oz | low-fat feta cheese, grated | 125 g |
| 8 | Greek black olives | 8 |
| 1 | lemon, cut in wedges (for garnish) | 1 |

**Dressing:**

| | | |
|---|---|---|
| 1 tbsp | olive oil | 15 mL |
| 2 tbsp | water | 25 mL |
| ¼ cup | lemon juice | 50 mL |
| 1 | clove garlic, minced | 1 |
| 1 tsp | dried oregano | 5 mL |
| | salt, black pepper (to taste) | |

1. In a large salad bowl, combine salad vegetables. Top with grated feta cheese and black olives. Garnish with lemon wedges.
2. In a small bowl, whisk together dressing. Toss with salad just before serving or serve dressing on the side.

Makes 4 servings.

# Summer's Here Pasta Salad

Make this quick and delicious pasta salad anytime you have leftover noodles. It's always a hit with my son Jason, especially in summer for backyard BBQ's. Toss in any veggies that you have on hand like peas, baby corn, broccoli, chickpeas or kidney beans. Almost any combination will work.

| | **The Lowdown** (per serving) | |
|---|---|---|
| calories | | 189 |
| fat | | 2 g |
| carbohydrate | | 36 g |
| protein | | 7 g |

| | | |
|---|---|---|
| 4 cups | rotini or penne pasta, cooked | 1 L |
| 1 cup | chickpeas (cooked or canned) | 250 mL |
| ½ each | green and red peppers, diced | ½ each |
| ¼ | English cucumber, chopped | ¼ |
| 1 | tomato, cubed | 1 |
| 2 tbsp | capers | 25 mL |
| | black pepper, (to taste) | |
| ½ cup | low-calorie or light Italian salad dressing | 125 mL |
| | black olives as garnish (optional) | |

1. In a large bowl combine cooked pasta, chickpeas, vegetables and capers. Season with fresh ground black pepper.
3. Toss with salad dressing. Cover and refrigerate for at least 2 hours.
4. Serve on a bed of salad greens garnished with black olives, if desired.

Makes 6 servings.

# Skinny Potato Salad

Your family won't miss the fat and calories when you serve them this trimmed down picnic favorite. You can use leftover potatoes if you have them and any other veggies you can think of.

| 2 lb | new potatoes, scrubbed, cooked until fork tender, cut in quarters | 1 kg |
|---|---|---|
| 1 | raw carrot, peeled and grated | 1 |
| 1 | celery stalk, diced | 1 |
| 2 | green onions, sliced | 2 |
| 2 tbsp | fresh parsley, chopped | 25 mL |

**Dressing:**

| ¼ cup | ultra-light or fat-free mayonnaise | 50 mL |
|---|---|---|
| 1 tsp | Dijon mustard | 5 mL |
| ½ tsp | salt (or to taste) | 2 mL |
| | freshly ground pepper (to taste) | |

1. In a large bowl combine cooled cooked potatoes, carrot, celery, green onions and parsley.
2. In a small bowl combine ultra-light mayonnaise and Dijon mustard.
3. Carefully add dressing to potatoes and vegetables.
4. Adjust seasonings, to taste. Cover and refrigerate until ready to serve.

Makes 8 servings.

# Oriental Slaw

Just in case you thought there were only two kinds of cole slaw, regular and creamy, here's a new one for you to try. Even Moishe at the deli will say it's okay. What could be bad?

| | | |
|---|---|---|
| 3 cups | red cabbage, shredded | 750 mL |
| 3 cups | green cabbage, shredded | 750 mL |
| 1 cup | carrots, scraped and shredded | 250 mL |
| 4 | green onions, thinly sliced | 4 |
| ¼ cup | raisins or dried cranberries | 50 mL |

**Dressing:**

| | | |
|---|---|---|
| 1 tbsp | sesame oil | 15 mL |
| ¼ cup | seasoned rice vinegar | 50 mL |
| ½ tsp | black pepper (to taste) | 2 mL |

**The Lowdown**
(per serving)

| | |
|---|---|
| calories | 60 |
| fat | 2 g |
| carbohydrate | 11 g |
| protein | 1 g |

1. In a large bowl, combine vegetables and raisins.
2. In a small bowl, whisk together dressing ingredients.
3. Add dressing to slaw and toss until well combined.
4. Cover and refrigerate for several hours or overnight.

Makes 8 servings.

# Bubie's Cucumber Salad

**The Lowdown**
(per serving)

| | |
|---|---|
| calories | 40 |
| fat | 0 g |
| carbohydrate | 9 g |
| protein | 1 g |

Bubie is my wonderful mother Pauline. Her traditional cucumber salad is always a hit at family gatherings. You can add grated carrot, onion and a few sprigs of dill, if you wish. Bubie makes it with just cucumbers and lots of love. And it's perfect.

| | | |
|---|---|---|
| 3 | cucumbers (12 oz / 375 g each), peeled and sliced in rounds | 3 |
| ½ tsp | salt | 2 mL |
| 1 cup | water | 250 mL |
| ⅓ cup | vinegar | 75 mL |
| 3 tbsp | white sugar (or equivalent sweetener) | 45 mL |
| ½ | grated carrot (optional) | ½ |
| ½ | onion, sliced in rings (optional) few sprigs fresh dill | ½ |

1. Place cucumber slices in a colander over a large bowl.
2. Sprinkle cucumber slices with salt. Make sure salt is well-distributed over the cucumber slices.
3. Cover cucumbers with plastic wrap and place a large can over the cucumbers as a weight. Allow to stand for about 3-4 hours.
4. Discard juice from cucumber slices. Rinse cucumber slices with water, and squeeze out excess water by hand.
5. Place squeezed cucumber slices in a clean glass bowl. Prepare dressing in a separate bowl and pour over cucumbers. Add grated carrot, onion and dill if using.
6. Cover bowl with plastic wrap and refrigerate overnight.

Makes 8 servings.

# El Rancho Creamy Dip

One summer, I whipped this up as a dip for veggies for a dinner party. No one ate the dip so I served it with the grilled salmon instead. It was outstanding. Everyone asked for my "sauce" recipe. Dip or sauce, it tastes great no matter what you call it.

| | | |
|---|---|---|
| 1 cup | fat-free sour cream | 250 mL |
| ¼ cup | ultra-light or fat-free mayonnaise | 50 mL |
| 2 tbsp | lemon juice | 25 mL |
| 1-2 | cloves garlic | 1-2 |
| ½ tsp | black pepper | 2 mL |
| ¼ cup | fresh dill | 50 mL |
| ½ tsp | salt (or to taste) | 2 mL |

**The Lowdown**
(per 1 tbsp / 15 mL)

| | |
|---|---|
| calories | 8 |
| fat | 0 g |
| carbohydrate | 2 g |
| protein | 1 g |

1. Place ingredients in food processor. Pulse on and off a few times until dressing is mixed.
2. Pour into a bowl, cover and chill in refrigerator until ready to use.

Makes about 1½ cups/375 mL dip.

# Creamy Eggplant and Vidalia Onion Dip

Serve as a dip with pita and veggies or as a side dish with fish, meat or chicken.

| | | |
|---|---|---|
| 1 | eggplant, sliced in rounds (about 1½ lb / 750 g) cooking spray | 1 |
| 1 | Vidalia or Spanish onion, peeled and sliced in rounds | 1 |
| 2 | cloves garlic, sliced fresh ground pepper (to taste) | 2 |
| ½ each | red and green pepper, seeded and cut in chunks | ½ each |
| 1 | tomato, diced | 1 |
| 2 tbsp | balsamic vinegar | 25 mL |
| ½ tsp | salt (or to taste) | 2 mL |
| 2 tbsp | ultra-light or fat-free mayonnaise few dashes hot pepper sauce (optional) | 25 mL |

1. Place sliced eggplant on a non-stick baking sheet. Top with sliced onion and garlic. Season with black pepper and spray lightly with cooking spray.
2. Bake for 35-40 minutes in a 325°F/160°C oven until eggplant, onion and garlic are soft. Remove from oven and allow to cool.
3. In bowl of food processor fitted with the steel blade, chop red and green pepper. Add cooled eggplant, onion and garlic, and pulse a few times until combined.
4. Add diced tomato, balsamic vinegar, salt, pepper, ultra-light mayonnaise and hot pepper sauce, to taste. Pulse a few times more until desired consistency is achieved.
5. Transfer mixture to a bowl, cover and refrigerate for at least 2 hours or overnight.

Makes 8 servings.

# Tzatziki with a Twist

This tzatziki tastes just like it came from Zorba's kitchen. Serve it as a dip with raw veggies, as a topping for baked potatoes or as a sauce for grilled chicken or fish. What's the twist, you ask? It's fat-free.

| | | |
|---|---|---|
| 1 cup | fat-free yogurt cheese | 250 mL |
| ½ cup | English cucumber, finely minced | 125 mL |
| 2 | cloves garlic, minced | 2 |
| 1 tbsp | lemon juice | 15 mL |
| 2 tbsp | fresh dill, chopped | 25 mL |
| ½ tsp | black pepper, salt (to taste) | 2 mL |

1. Combine ingredients and mix well. Pour into a small bowl, cover and refrigerate until ready to serve.

Makes 1½ cups/375 mL.

# Sharon's Vinaigrette

This was one of my first recipes and is still a favorite. Use it as a basic vinaigrette with almost any combination of oil and vinegar. Olive oil and balsamic vinegar make a great paring, as do sunflower oil and red wine vinegar. What's important is the proportion to keep fat and calories light.

| | | |
|---|---|---|
| 2 tbsp | oil | 25 mL |
| 2 tbsp | water | 25 mL |
| ½ cup | vinegar | 125 mL |
| 2 tsp | sugar or equivalent sweetener | 10 mL |
| ½ tsp | salt (or to taste) | 2 mL |
| ½ tsp | garlic powder | 2 mL |
| ½ tsp | black pepper (or to taste) | 2 mL |

1. Combine ingredients in a measuring cup. Stir vigorously to combine thoroughly.

Makes ¾ cup/175 mL dressing.

# Cool as A Cucumber Creamy Dressing

Love that creamy taste but hate the fat and calories? This makes a yummy substitute.

| | | |
|---|---|---|
| 1 cup | plain fat-free yogurt | 250 mL |
| ¼ | English cucumber, peeled and sliced in chunks | ¼ |
| ¼ | red onion, chopped | ¼ |
| 1-2 | cloves garlic | 1-2 |
| ¼ cup | fresh dill | 50 mL |
| ½ tsp | salt (or to taste) | 2 mL |
| ¼ tsp | pepper (or to taste) | 1 mL |

**The Lowdown**
(per 1 tbsp / 15 mL)

| | |
|---|---|
| calories | 6 |
| fat | 0 g |
| carbohydrate | 1 g |
| protein | 1 g |

1. Purée ingredients in food processor or blender.
2. Serve over salad greens, cucumber, tomato, onion, green and red pepper.

Makes 1½ cup / 375 mL dressing.

# Cranberry Vinaigrette

Cranberry juice on a salad? The color is gorgeous and the taste divine. Delicious over mixed greens with grilled chicken, or tossed with spinach, sliced mushrooms, water chestnuts, bean sprouts and grated hard-boiled egg whites.

| | | |
|---|---|---|
| ⅔ cup | cranberry juice cocktail | 150 mL |
| ¼ cup | red wine vinegar | 50 mL |
| 1 oz | red onion | 25 g |
| ½ tsp | salt | 2 mL |
| ¼ tsp | black pepper | 1 mL |
| ¼ tsp | garlic powder | 1 mL |
| 1 tsp | dried tarragon | 5 mL |
| 1 tsp | dried thyme | 5 mL |

1. Place ingredients in bowl of food processor fitted with steel blade. Process until onion is finely minced.

Makes 1 cup/250 mL dressing.

# Citrus Vinaigrette

This dressing is wonderful over mixed greens and slices of grilled tuna or chicken. The onion combined with the orange juice, rice vinegar and garlic will perk up your tastebuds.

| | | |
|---|---|---|
| 2 oz | red or white onion, cut in chunks | 50 g |
| 1 | clove garlic, sliced | 1 |
| ⅔ cup | orange juice | 150 mL |
| ¼ cup | seasoned rice vineger | 50 mL |
| ½ tsp | black pepper (or to taste) | 2 mL |

1. Place onion and garlic in bowl of food processor fitted with the steel blade. Process until minced.
2. Add orange juice, vinegar and black pepper.
3. Process until ingredients are well-combined.
4. Pour into a small bowl.
5. Cover and refrigerate until ready to serve.

Makes 1 cup / 250 mL dressing.

# Mango Salsa

**The Lowdown**
(per 1 tbsp / 15 mL)

| | |
|---|---|
| calories | 8 |
| fat | 0 g |
| carbohydrates | 2 g |
| protein | 0 g |

**Highlight**

To cut your mango, first peel it with a potato peeler, then cut thick slices off the pit. You can then slice and dice your mango with ease.

Serve this lovely salsa with grilled chicken or fish. If you like to turn up the heat, add a drop or two of hot pepper sauce. If not, leave it out. It will taste great either way.

| | | |
|---|---|---|
| 1 | mango, peeled and diced | 1 |
| ½ | red bell pepper, seeded and diced | ½ |
| ½ | green sweet banana pepper, seeded and diced | ½ |
| 3 tbsp | red onion, finely chopped | 45 mL |
| 1 tbsp | chopped cilantro or parsley | 15 mL |
| 1 tbsp | seasoned rice vinegar | 15 mL |
| 1-2 drops | hot pepper sauce (optional) | 1-2 drops |

1. Combine ingredients in a small bowl.
2. Cover and refrigerate until ready to serve.

Makes about 1½ cups / 375 mL salsa.

# CHAPTER 13

# *Soup-er Soups*

$S$OUPS FOR ALL SEASONS, soups for all reasons. On a cold winter's day, there's nothing like a steaming bowl of vegetable soup to satisfy a hearty appetite and warm the soul. On a hot day, a bowl of chilled gazpacho is a great way to stay cool, calm and collected.

When I started creating the soup recipes, I was delighted to see how beneficial they were in helping my clients achieve their healthy eating goals. So I kept the soup recipes coming. One January, when I was asked in an interview for a New Year's healthy eating tip, I had a one-word answer, "Soup!"

Most soups, other than cream soups, are generally low in fat, have a high water content, and usually contain vegetables. This makes soup low in calories and filling at the same time. Have we died and gone to heaven? Low calorie food that is filling and satisfying too. No wonder I call soup your secret weapon in winning the battle of the belly.

Not only will soup help trim your waistline, eating soup can also help transform your eating habits. You can't gulp hot soup quickly or you'll burn your mouth. That hurts! You have to eat soup sitting at a table or you'll spill all over yourself. What a mess! You can't do other things while you're eating soup so you'll actually get to enjoy what you're eating.

> *On a cold winter's day, there's nothing like a steaming bowl of vegetable soup to satisfy a hearty appetite and warm the soul.*

Start making these soups for yourself and see what I mean. You'll get hooked before you know it. Soon soup will be a must on your healthy eating plan too.

This is what my clients do. They make a new batch of soup each week. That way they can have a bowl of soup ready to enjoy with a sandwich for lunch, to zap in the microwave as a snack until supper's ready, and before they go out to a party, they enjoy a mug of soup and a cracker so they won't be tempted to overeat later on. If it's there in the refrigerator, ready and waiting, soup can be your secret weapon in achieving your healthy eating goals too.

## Soup-er Tips

1. Soften onion and garlic in a little water instead of oil to cut down on fat.

2. Add a potato or two to thicken your soup. The added calories are worth it and can be counted as part of a starch serving.

3. Always make ahead and chill soups containing meat ingredients so that the hardened fat can be removed before serving.

4. For a protein boost, add canned chickpeas, beans or lentils to turn your soup into a complete meal.

5. If adding canned ingredients to your soup, rinse whenever possible and use very little, if any salt.

6. Be daring when making soups. A variety of vegetables, herbs and spices, lemon juice or vinegar, Worcestershire or hot pepper sauce can perk up almost any soup.

7. If soup is too thick, add a little water or broth. If too thin, add a potato, rice or pasta to thicken.

*Always make ahead and chill soups containing meat ingredients so that the hardened fat can be removed before serving.*

8. Save cooking water from boiling potatoes or steaming vegetables to be used as a vegetable stock for soup instead of water.

9. To purée soups with ease, invest in a hand-held purée wand that goes right into the soup pot. It saves alot of mess and hassle when you want to blend your soup.

10. Whenever a recipe calls for defatted chicken broth, you can refrigerate chicken broth overnight and remove all traces of hardened fat. Or use canned fat-free chicken broth diluted with water.

11. The soup recipes generally make large batches, about eight to ten servings. If you know you won't use it all, you can either make half the recipe or take turns making the soups with a friend and take half each. Or you can freeze some. Most of the soups, except for the gazpacho and the cabbage soup, freeze well.

12. Cilantro is also called Chinese parsley. It has a very distinctive taste. If you or your family dislike it, you can substitute curly or Italian broad-leafed parsley in the recipes. Or you can try to develop a taste for it. It will be worth it.

*If you know you won't use it all, you can either make half the recipe or take turns making the soups with a friend and take half each.*

# Soup Recipes

# Zero Zucchini Soup

Quick and extra-easy, this puréed soup has a lovely texture. The zero stands for zero added fat.

| | | |
|---|---|---|
| 8 | large zucchini, cut in chunks | 8 |
| 4 | carrots, peeled and sliced | 4 |
| 1 | onion, chopped | 1 |
| 1 | potato, peeled and cut in pieces | 1 |
| | water, to cover | |
| 2 tbsp | parsley, chopped | 25 mL |
| 2 tbsp | low-sodium chicken-flavored soup mix | 25 mL |
| 1-2 tsp | dried tarragon | 5-10 mL |
| ½ tsp | black pepper (or to taste) | 2 mL |
| | salt (to taste) | |

**The Lowdown**
(per serving)

| | |
|---|---|
| calories | 60 |
| fat | 1 g |
| carbohydrate | 12 g |
| protein | 3 g |

1. Place first four ingredients in a large soup pot.
2. Add water to cover and bring to a boil.
3. Reduce heat and add remaining ingredients.
4. Simmer on low heat for 30 minutes or until vegetables are cooked and soft. Adjust seasonings, to taste.
5. Allow soup to cool. Purée in a blender, food processor or with a hand-held blender. Reheat to serve.

Makes 8 servings.

# Curried Squash Soup

You'll want to serve this lovely soup any time, or when you have guests for dinner. Just dress it up with a dollop of fat-free sour cream and a few long chives criss-crossed on top.

| | | |
|---|---|---|
| 2 lb | butternut squash, cut in small pieces | 1 kg |
| 1 | Spanish onion, chopped | 1 |
| 2 | carrots, peeled and sliced | 2 |
| 1 | Spy apple, cored, peeled and chopped | 1 |
| 1 | potato, peeled and chopped | 1 |
| 4 cups | defatted chicken broth | 1 L |
| ½ cup | orange juice | 125 mL |
| ½ tsp | nutmeg (or to taste) | 2 mL |
| ½ tsp | cinnamon (or to taste) | 2 mL |
| ½ tsp | allspice (or to taste) | 2 mL |
| 1 tbsp | curry powder (or to taste) | 15 mL |
| | salt and pepper (to taste) | |
| | fat-free sour cream (optional) | |
| | chives (optional) | |

1. Combine all ingredients, except sour cream and chives, in a large soup pot. Bring to a boil and simmer gently for 1 hour, or until vegetables are soft.
2. When cooled, purée soup in a blender, food processor or with a hand-held blender.
3. If soup is too thin, simmer uncovered for a few minutes to thicken soup. If soup is too thick, add additional broth. Adjust seasonings, to taste.
4. To serve, reheat soup thoroughly.

Makes 10 servings.

# Squash and Chickpea Soup

This thick and flavorful soup is brimming with the anti-oxidant beta-carotene. The chickpeas add a boost of protein. To save preparation time, use butternut squash that has already been peeled and cubed.

| | | |
|---|---|---|
| 1 | onion, chopped | 1 |
| 1 lb | butternut squash, cubed | 500 g |
| 1 | 19 oz / 540 mL can chickpeas, drained and rinsed | 1 |
| 4 cups | defatted chicken broth or water black pepper (to taste) | 1 L |
| 2 tbsp | parsley or cilantro, chopped | 25 mL |
| 1 tbsp | curry powder (optional) | 15 mL |

1. In a large non-stick pot cook onion in a little water until softened.
2. Add remaining ingredients, bring to a boil, reduce heat and simmer covered for about 1½ hours or until vegetables are soft.
3. Allow soup to cool. Purée soup in a blender, food processor or with a hand-held blender. Adjust seasonings, to taste.
4. Reheat soup before serving.

Makes 8 servings.

**The Lowdown**
(per serving)

| | |
|---|---|
| calories | 86 |
| fat | 1 g |
| carbohydrate | 15 g |
| protein | 4 g |

# Guilt-Free Cauliflower Soup

Rich and creamy, just like the decadent cauliflower soup made with cream, but with a fraction of the fat and calories.

**The Lowdown**
(per serving)

| | | |
|---|---|---:|
| calories | | 51 |
| fat | | 0 g |
| carbohydrate | | 10 g |
| protein | | 3 g |

| | | |
|---|---|---|
| 1 | head cauliflower, cut in florets | 1 |
| 1 | onion, chopped | 1 |
| 2 | cloves garlic, minced | 2 |
| 4 | carrots, peeled and sliced | 4 |
| 2 | potatoes, peeled and cut in quarters | 2 |
| 6 cups | defatted chicken broth | 1.5 L |
| 2 tbsp | chopped parsley | 25 mL |
| | salt and pepper, to taste | |
| 1 tbsp | curry powder (optional) | 15 mL |

1. In a large non-stick soup pot, cook onion and garlic in a little water until softened.
2. Add remaining ingredients.
3. Bring to a boil, reduce heat and simmer covered for 1 hour, or until vegetables are soft.
4. Allow soup to cool. Purée soup in a blender, food processor or with a hand-held blender. Adjust seasonings, to taste.
5. Reheat soup before serving.

Makes 12 servings.

# California Dreamin' Vegetable Soup

This is a variation of the Guilt-Free Cauliflower Soup. One winter when the price of fresh cauliflower went sky high, a savvy client suggested using frozen California vegetables to make this soup. It was a great tip. Thanks!

| | | |
|---|---|---|
| 2 lb | frozen California-style vegetables (broccoli, cauliflower, carrots) | 1 kg |
| 1 | onion, chopped | 1 |
| 2 | cloves garlic, minced | 2 |
| 2 | potatoes, peeled and cubed | 2 |
| 6 cups | defatted chicken broth or water | 1.5 L |
| 2 tbsp | parsley, chopped | 25 mL |
| ½ tsp | dried tarragon | 2 mL |
| ½ tsp | dried dill | 2 mL |
| | salt and pepper (to taste) | |
| 1 tbsp | curry powder (optional) | 15 mL |

1. In a large non-stick soup pot, cook onion and garlic in a little water until softened.
2. Add remaining ingredients.
3. Bring to a boil, reduce heat, and simmer covered for 1 hour or until vegetables are soft.
4. Allow soup to cool. Purée soup in a blender, food processor or with a hand-held blender. Adjust seasonings, to taste.
5. Reheat soup before serving.

Makes 10 servings.

# Mushroom Barley Potage

Mushrooms and barley combine to create a thick and hearty soup that not only tastes great but is good for you too. Barley is a good source of soluble fiber, which helps to reduce cholesterol, stabilize blood sugars and prevent constipation.

**The Lowdown**
(per serving)

| | |
|---|---|
| calories | 66 |
| fat | 0 g |
| carbohydrate | 13 g |
| protein | 4 g |

| | | |
|---|---|---|
| 1 | onion, chopped | 1 |
| 1 | clove garlic, minced | 1 |
| 1 | large carrot, peeled and sliced | 1 |
| 1 | celery stalk, sliced | 1 |
| 1 lb | mushrooms (white, shiitake, portobello), sliced | 500 g |
| ½ cup | pearl barley, rinsed | 125 mL |
| 6 cups | defatted chicken broth | 1.5 L |
| 2 tbsp | parsley, chopped | 25 mL |
| 1 tsp | salt (or to taste) | 5 mL |
| 1 tsp | black pepper (or to taste) | 5 mL |

1. In a large non-stick soup pot, cook onion and garlic in a little water on medium heat.
2. Add carrots, celery, mushrooms and about one cup/250 mL chicken broth. Continue cooking for about 5 minutes, or until mushrooms are softened.
3. Add barley, remaining chicken broth and seasonings. Stir to combine.
4. Reduce heat, cover and simmer for 1 hour. Adjust seasonings to taste.
5. Reheat before serving.

Makes 10 servings.

# Magic Minestrone

When my dear Dad was recovering from an illness a while ago, he said that he'd love to have a bowl of minestrone soup. So we made him this soup. He enjoyed it so much, he ate it every day for lunch. He got better and I started calling it "Magic Minestrone".

**The Lowdown**
(per serving)

| | |
|---|---|
| calories | 103 |
| fat | 0 g |
| carbohydrate | 21 g |
| protein | 4 g |

| | | |
|---|---|---|
| 1 | onion, chopped | 1 |
| 1-2 | cloves garlic, minced | 1-2 |
| 2 | carrots, peeled and sliced | 2 |
| 1 | celery stalk, sliced | 1 |
| 1 | parsnip, peeled and sliced | 1 |
| 1 | 28 oz / 796 mL can plum or crushed tomatoes | 1 |
| 2 | potatoes, peeled and diced | 2 |
| 4 cups | water | 1 L |
| ¼ cup | fresh parsley, chopped | 50 mL |
| 1 cup | canned kidney beans, rinsed | 250 mL |
| ½ cup | small pasta noodles (uncooked) | 125 mL |
| 1 tsp | Italian seasoning | 5 mL |
| | black pepper (to taste) | |

1. In a non-stick soup pot, cook onion and garlic in a little water on medium-high heat.
2. Add carrots, celery, parsnip and a small amount of water, and continue to cook vegetables for a few minutes.
3. Add potatoes, tomatoes, parsley, and 4 cups/1 L water (or enough to cover vegetables). Bring to a boil and simmer on low heat for 30 minutes.
4. Add pasta and continue to simmer for 15 minutes more, until pasta is cooked.
5. Add kidney beans, adjust seasonings and simmer on low heat until ready to serve.

Makes 10 servings.

# Lentil Salsa Soup

Even mild salsa can taste super-spicy when it is heated, so you may want to experiment with how much you use in this soup.

**The Lowdown**
(per serving)

| | |
|---|---|
| calories | 114 |
| fat | 0 g |
| carbohydrate | 22 g |
| protein | 6 g |

| | | |
|---|---|---|
| 1 | medium onion, chopped | 1 |
| 1-2 | cloves garlic, minced | 1-2 |
| 2 | medium carrots, peeled and sliced | 2 |
| 2 | celery stalks, sliced | 2 |
| 1 cup | chunky salsa (mild) | 250 mL |
| 1 | 28 oz/796 mL can stewed tomatoes | 1 |
| 1 | 19 oz/540 mL can lentils, drained and rinsed | 1 |
| 2 cups | water | 500 mL |
| 2 tbsp | parsley, chopped | 25 mL |
| | black pepper, (to taste) | |

1. In a non-stick soup pot, cook chopped onion and garlic in a little water. Add carrots and celery and continue to cook until vegetables are softened.
2. Add lentils, stewed tomatoes, water, salsa, parsley, and black pepper. Stir to combine.
3. Bring to a boil. Reduce heat and simmer covered for about 30 minutes or until carrots are cooked. Stir occasionally.

Makes 8 servings.

# Farmer's Market Vegetable Soup

All the goodness of a farmer's market packed into a bowl. Add a slice or two of whole grain bread, and a bowl of fresh fruit and yogurt for dessert.

<table>
<tr><td>1</td><td>onion, chopped</td><td>1</td></tr>
<tr><td>2</td><td>cloves garlic, minced</td><td>2</td></tr>
<tr><td>3</td><td>celery stalks, sliced</td><td>3</td></tr>
<tr><td>3</td><td>carrots, peeled and sliced</td><td>3</td></tr>
<tr><td>1</td><td>potato, peeled and cubed</td><td>1</td></tr>
<tr><td>1</td><td>parsnip, peeled and diced</td><td>1</td></tr>
<tr><td>½ cup</td><td>water</td><td>125 mL</td></tr>
<tr><td>1</td><td>48 oz/1.36 L can vegetable juice cocktail</td><td>1</td></tr>
<tr><td>2 tbsp</td><td>parsley, chopped</td><td>25 mL</td></tr>
<tr><td></td><td>black pepper, (to taste)</td><td></td></tr>
<tr><td>dash</td><td>Worcestershire sauce</td><td>dash</td></tr>
<tr><td>½ cup</td><td>frozen peas</td><td>125 mL</td></tr>
<tr><td>½ cup</td><td>frozen corn niblets</td><td>125 mL</td></tr>
</table>

**The Lowdown**
(per serving)

| | |
|---|---|
| calories | 74 |
| fat | 0 g |
| carbohydrate | 17 g |
| protein | 2 g |

1. In a large non-stick soup pot, cook onion, garlic, celery, carrots, and parsnip in ½ cup/125 mL water, stirring well. Cover and cook over low heat for 10 minutes, stirring occasionally.
2. Add vegetable juice cocktail, parsley, potato and seasonings. Stir, bring to a boil, and simmer over low heat for 20 minutes until vegetables are tender.
3. Add peas and corn, and simmer for 10 minutes more.

Makes 8 servings.

# Chicken Soup for The Healthy Eater's Soul

This is the real thing! Enjoy with rice, noodles or a matzo ball. The addition of a turkey part provides a deep, rich flavor.

| | | |
|---|---|---|
| 1 | chicken carcass | 1 |
| 1 | turkey wing or drumstick | 1 |
| 8 cups | water | 2 L |
| 4 | carrots, peeled | 4 |
| 2 | parsnips, peeled | 2 |
| 2 | celery stalks and leaves, chopped | 2 |
| 1 | onion, peeled and quartered | 1 |
| 2 tbsp | chopped parsley | 25 mL |
| 1 tsp | salt (or to taste) | 5 mL |

1. Place chicken carcass, turkey part and water in a large soup pot and bring to a boil.
2. Skim to remove foam which forms and rises to the top.
3. Add remaining ingredients and continue to skim until no foam continues to form.
4. Cover pot and simmer on low heat for approximately 1½ hours.
5. Strain soup in a colander. Reserve turkey meat for sandwiches or to toss into a salad.
6. Refrigerate soup overnight to allow fat to harden on the surface.
7. Remove hardened fat from the surface of the soup.
8. Reheat and serve.

Makes 8 servings.

# Tomato Cabbage Borscht

This isn't the soup from the "cabbage soup diet", but it can still give you a headstart on achieving your healthy weight and eating goals. And your family will like it too.

**The Lowdown**
(per serving)

| | |
|---|---|
| calories | 69 |
| fat | 0 g |
| carbohydrate | 16 g |
| protein | 2 g |

| | | |
|---|---|---|
| 1 | onion, chopped | 1 |
| 2 | carrots, peeled and sliced in rounds | 2 |
| 1 | celery stalk, sliced | 1 |
| 1 lb | cabbage, shredded | 500 g |
| 1 | 28 oz / 796 mL can crushed tomatoes | 1 |
| 4 cups | water | 1 L |
| ½ tsp | black pepper | 2 mL |
| ¼ cup | sugar or equivalent sweetener (or to taste) | 50 mL |
| 2 | bay leaves | 2 |
| 1 tsp | Worcestershire sauce | 5 mL |
| 2 tbsp | chopped parsley | 25 mL |
| | juice of ½ a lemon | |

1. Cook onion, carrots and celery in ½ cup / 125 mL water in a large non-stick soup pot.
2. Add cabbage, tomatoes, and water. Cover pot and bring to a boil.
3. Add remaining ingredients. Reduce heat and simmer for approximately 1½ hours, or until cabbage is soft. Adjust seasonings, to taste.
4. When soup is ready, remove and discard bay leaves.

Makes 10 servings.

# Broccoli and Potato Soup

This is an easy way to get your family to eat broccoli, which in my opinion, is the superstar of vegetables.

**The Lowdown**
(per serving)

| | |
|---|---|
| calories | 50 |
| fat | 0 g |
| carbohydrate | 10 g |
| protein | 3 g |

| | | |
|---|---|---|
| 1 | large Spanish onion, chopped | 1 |
| 1 | bunch broccoli, stems peeled and chopped, reserve broccoli florets | 1 |
| 2 | potatoes, peeled and chopped | 2 |
| 2 | carrots, peeled and sliced in rounds | 2 |
| 6 cups | defatted chicken broth | 1.5 L |
| 2 tbsp | chopped parsley | 25 mL |
| | salt, pepper (to taste) | |

1. Combine onion, chopped broccoli, carrot, potato and chicken broth in a large non-stick soup pot and bring to a boil.
2. Reduce heat, add parsley, salt and pepper, to taste. Simmer, covered for approximately 30-40 minutes, or until vegetables are soft.
3. Allow soup to cool. Purée soup in a blender, food processor or with a hand-held blender.
4. Before serving, reheat soup and bring to a slow bowl. Add reserved broccoli florets and simmer for approximately 5 minutes. Adjust seasonings, to taste.

Makes 10 servings.

# Stay Cool Creamy Gazpacho

This is your summertime salvation. While everyone else is tucking into their chilled cream soups, you can keep cool and trim with this low-cal wonder. The yogurt turns your gazpacho a pretty shade of pink.

| | The Lowdown (per serving) | |
|---|---|---|
| calories | | 54 |
| fat | | 0 g |
| carbohydrate | | 11 g |
| protein | | 3 g |

| | | |
|---|---|---|
| 1 | onion, peeled and quartered | 1 |
| ½ | English cucumber, not peeled, cut in chunks | ½ |
| ½ each | red and green peppers, seeded and cut in chunks | ½ each |
| 1½ cups | plain fat-free yogurt | 375 mL |
| 1 | 48 oz / 1.36 L can tomato juice | 1 |
| 2 tbsp | chopped fresh cilantro or parsley or 1 tsp (5 mL) dried black pepper (to taste) croutons (for garnish) | 25 mL |

1. In food processor fitted with the steel blade, mince onion. Add cucumber and red and green peppers. Process until vegetables are chopped.
2. Transfer vegetables to a large bowl. Stir in tomato juice, cilantro and black pepper.
3. Add yogurt and stir until thoroughly combined.
4. Cover and chill in refrigerator overnight.
5. Serve cold garnished with croutons, if desired.

Makes 10 servings.

# CHAPTER 14

# *Veggies are Vital*

VEGETABLES ARE PLAYING a more important role in the way we eat. After years of taking a back seat to the heftier items on the plate like meats and starches, vegetables are finally getting the respect they deserve. And for good reason.

Think of vegetables as your nutritional super-heroes. They're loaded with vitamins, minerals, protective phyto-chemicals that help fight disease, anti-oxidants that neutral-ize free radicals in the body, fiber and even water. And they're naturally low in fat and calories. Vegetables are your best allies to help you achieve your healthy weight and lifestyle goals. I hope you'll never think of them as skimpy side-dishes again.

When Canada's Food Guide was revised, the "Fruits and Vegetables" food group was renamed "Vegetables and Fruits". To me, this emphasizes how important vegetables truly are. Perhaps we'll see the old adage "an apple a day" become "a serving of broccoli a day" sometime soon.

Along with their nutritional benefits, vegetables are also wonderfully diverse and delicious. Just the way salad can double as a complete meal, other vegetables have become main course players too. They figure prominently in stir-fries, chilis and pasta dishes. The protein part of the meal

*They're loaded with vitamins, minerals, protective phytochemicals that help fight disease, anti-oxidants that neutralize free radicals in the body, fiber and even water.*

can easily be provided by plant-based choices like chickpeas, beans, lentils or tofu instead of meat, chicken or fish.

Of course, you can still enjoy your veggies as a side dish. But the difference is that instead of taking up a mere quarter of the plate as before, today they're staking their claim to at least half the plate or more.

Starchy vegetables like potatoes, winter squash and corn can be higher in calories, so count them as a starch serving. Balance them with lighter choices like cauliflower, zucchini, mushrooms and green beans. Be sure to go for deep-colored green and orange vegetables whenever possible. They tend to be the most nutritious.

*Starchy vegetables like potatoes, winter squash and corn can be higher in calories, so count them as a starch serving.*

## Veggie Vitals

1. Use Yukon golds for mashed potatoes. They have a naturally buttery taste and appearance. Cook with a clove or two or more of garlic and mash with reserved cooking water. You won't miss the butter and cream.

2. Steam or microwave fresh veggies for a short time with a minimum of water to retain nutrients, taste and texture.

3. After you've had oven "fried" potatoes, you'll never want their greasy cousins. Spray a non-stick baking sheet with cooking spray. Use new, red or baking potatoes cut into strips with skin on for best results.

4. Oven-ready noodles for vegetarian lasagna need plenty of liquid to cook properly. The veggies in the lasagna recipe help by giving off water which is absorbed by the noodles.

5. For convenience, use canned dried beans as a good alternative to soaking and cooking your own. Be sure to drain and rinse with water to remove excess salt.

# Vegetable Recipes

# Speedy Vegetarian Chili

This is the recipe that got me started. A friend told me that after all these years, she still makes this chili for family and friends and it's always a hit. I hope it will be with you and yours too.

| | | |
|---|---|---|
| 1 | onion, chopped | 1 |
| ½ lb | mushrooms, sliced | 250 g |
| 1 | carrot, peeled and sliced | 1 |
| 1 | celery stalk, sliced | 1 |
| ½ each | green and red pepper, seeded and chopped | ½ each |
| 1 | 19 oz / 540 mL can red kidney beans, drained and rinsed | 1 |
| 1 | 19 oz / 540 mL can chickpeas, drained and rinsed | 1 |
| 1 | 28 oz / 796 mL can stewed, diced or crushed tomatoes | 1 |
| 1 tsp | ground cumin | 5 mL |
| 1-2 tbsp | chili powder (or to taste) | 15-25 mL |
| 2 tbsp | chopped parsley | 25 mL |

**The Lowdown**
(per serving)

| | |
|---|---|
| calories | 240 |
| fat | 4 g |
| carbohydrates | 43 g |
| protein | 11 g |

1. In a non-stick pot, cook onion in a little water until softened.
2. Add mushrooms and continue cooking for about 5 minutes. Add carrot, celery, green and red pepper. Combine well.
3. Add beans, chickpeas, tomatoes and seasonings, to taste.
4. Add chopped parsley and stir.
5. Simmer covered for about 30 minutes or until vegetables are tender, stirring occasionally.

Makes 6 servings.

# Tofu Lasagna

If you've never cooked with tofu or dreamed of putting it in a lasagna, you've got to try this recipe. It's absolutely delicious, low in fat, and super-simple to make. When my daughter Leslie is home from university, we make this lasagna together, at least once or twice a week.

| | | |
|---|---|---|
| 16 oz | soft tofu, drained | 500 g |
| 2 | egg whites or ¼ cup/50 mL egg whites in a carton, lightly beaten | 2 |
| 2 tbsp | grated Parmesan cheese | 25 mL |
| ½ tsp | black pepper | 2 mL |
| ½ tsp | garlic powder | 2 mL |
| ½ lb | mushrooms, sliced | 250 g |
| 1 | zucchini, grated | 1 |
| 9 | oven-ready lasagna noodles | 9 |
| 3 cups | pasta sauce (meatless) | 750 mL |
| 6 oz | part-skim Mozzarella cheese, shredded | 175 g |

1. In a bowl, mash tofu with egg whites, pepper, garlic powder and 1 tbsp/15 mL grated Parmesan cheese. Set aside.
2. In an oblong lasagna pan, spoon 1 cup/250 mL sauce over bottom. Place 3 lasagna noodles on sauce, spread tofu mixture over noodles, and top with 3 more noodles.
3. Spread 1 cup/250 mL sauce over noodles. Top sauce with shredded Mozzarella cheese.
4. Place sliced mushrooms and zucchini in a single layer over cheese. Top with last 3 noodles.
5. Spread remaining sauce over final noodle layer. Sprinkle with 1 tbsp/15 mL grated Parmesan cheese.
6. Cover pan with foil. Bake in a 375°F/190°C oven for 1½ hours.
7. Remove lasagna from oven and allow to rest for 15 minutes before cutting.

Makes 8 servings.

# Last-Minute Lasagna

You just got a phone call from your hubby. Some friends are in town. He's invited them to come over for supper so they can see the kids. Do you (A) panic (B) order in, or (C) throw together this delicious lasagna, pop it in the oven and then sit back and enjoy the compliments. This recipe is an example of what you can do with a few pantry staples and some veggies that you keep on hand. P.S. I hope you choose (C). It's definitely the best answer.

| | | |
|---|---|---|
| 1 | small onion, chopped | 1 |
| ½ each | red and green pepper, seeded and chopped | ½ each |
| 1 | zucchini, grated | 1 |
| ½ lb | white mushrooms, sliced | 250 g |
| 1-2 | cloves garlic, minced | 1-2 |
| 2 cups | 1% cottage cheese | 500 mL |
| 2 | egg whites or ¼ cup/50 mL egg whites in a carton, lightly beaten | 2 |
| 3 cups | pasta sauce (meatless) | 750 mL |
| 9 | oven-ready lasagna noodles | 9 |
| 6 oz | part-skim Mozzarella cheese, shredded | 175 g |
| 2 tbsp | grated Parmesan cheese | 25 mL |

1. In a large non-stick pan, cook onion and garlic in a little water on medium-high heat until softened.
2. Add red and green pepper, zucchini and mushrooms. Season with black pepper, to taste. Continue to cook until vegetables are softened. Add a little water as needed. Set aside.
3. In a small bowl, combine cottage cheese with egg whites and 1 tbsp/15 mL grated Parmesan cheese. Set aside.

## The Lowdown
(per serving)

| | |
|---|---|
| calories | 246 |
| fat | 3g |
| carbohydrates | 39g |
| protein | 15g |

## Highlight

Have Hubby pick up a loaf of crusty Italian bread and some low-fat frozen yogurt to serve with fresh fruit for dessert. Break open that bag of washed salad greens that you keep in the vegetable drawer. Toss it with light Italian dressing or Sharon's Vinaigrette, with some oregano and basil mixed in. Or defrost some leftover Magic Minestrone that you have in the freezer. Lastly, if you don't have any fresh vegetables for the lasagna, use frozen Italian veggies that are just perfect at a time like this.

4. In a lasagna pan, spoon 1 cup/250 mL sauce over bottom. Place 3 lasagna noodles over sauce.

4. Spoon cottage cheese mixture over layer of noodles. Cover with a layer of 3 noodles.

5. Spoon 1 cup/250 mL of sauce over noodles. Top noodles with shredded Mozzarella cheese. Spread softened vegetables over cheese. Cover with remaining 3 noodles.

6. Spoon remaining sauce over noodles to cover. Sprinkle with grated 1 tbsp/15 mL Parmesan cheese.

7. Cover lasagna with foil. Bake in a 375°F/190°C oven for 1 hour.

8. Remove lasagna from oven and allow to rest for 15 minutes before cutting

Makes 8 servings.

# Presto Pasta Primavera

If you don't have time to go shopping for fresh vegetables, no problem. Just toss a few cups of frozen Italian mixed veggies into the sauce while your pasta is cooking. Presto, pasta primavera.

| | | |
|---|---|---|
| 1 | onion, chopped | 1 |
| 2 | cloves garlic, minced | 2 |
| ½ each | red, yellow and green peppers, seeded and thinly sliced | ½ each |
| ½ lb | mushrooms, sliced | 250 g |
| 1 | zucchini, sliced in rounds | 1 |
| 2 tbsp | chopped fresh basil or 1 tsp/5 mL dried | 25 mL |
| 3 cups | pasta sauce (meatless) | 750 mL |
| ½ lb | penne or other short pasta | 250 g |
| 2 tbsp | grated Parmesan cheese hot pepper flakes (optional) | 25 mL |

1. In a non-stick pot, cook onion and garlic in a little water until softened.
2. Add remaining vegetables and continue to cook for a few minutes more. Add pasta sauce and basil. Simmer covered until sauce is heated through.
3. Bring large pot of water to a boil. Add penne pasta and cook until tender but firm. Drain pasta.
4. To serve, place one cup/250 mL pasta on plate. Top with sauce and sprinkle with grated Parmesan cheese. Season with hot pepper flakes, if desired.

Makes 4 servings.

# "Beautiful You" Tofu Stir-Fry

I once appeared in a TV segment on "Beauty Foods". First we went to a food market where I pointed out 10 foods that might contribute to beauty and health. Then I cooked a "Beauty Foods" lunch. This simple stir-fry was the main course. When we were finished shooting, the crew and I sat down to eat what I had cooked. To my delight, my stir-fry which looked great on camera, tasted as good as it looked!

| | cooking spray | |
|---|---|---|
| 16 oz | firm tofu, cut in cubes | 500 g |
| 1 tsp | minced ginger | 5 mL |
| 1 tsp | minced garlic | 5 mL |
| 4 cups | frozen Oriental-style vegetables | 1 L |
| 2 tbsp | low-sodium soy sauce | 25 mL |
| 1 tsp | sesame oil | 5 mL |

1. Spray a large non-stick pan or wok with cooking spray. Lightly stir-fry tofu cubes with ginger and garlic over medium-high heat. Add a little water if tofu starts to stick to the pan.
2. Add frozen vegetables, soy sauce and sesame oil. Continue to stir-fry until vegetables are just cooked. Serve immediately.

Makes 4 servings.

# "Beauty" Foods

Although we really don't know for sure, the following may contribute to a beautiful appearance for the reasons given. In any case, feel beautiful about yourself for seeing the light and eating in a healthy way.

1. Water helps keep skin cells hydrated and flushes out impurities from the body.

2. Broccoli is rich in phytochemicals (plant compounds) that help our bodies fight disease and protect skin cells from oxidative damage.

3. Carrots and other orange vegetables and fruit are brimming with beta-carotene, an anti-oxidant that converts to vitamin A, essential for healthy hair, skin, eyes and mucous membranes.

4. Citrus fruits like oranges, grapefruit, tangerines, and lemons are rich in vitamin C, an important anti-oxidant which protects cells from oxidative damage and premature ageing.

5. Skim milk, fat-free yogurt and low-fat cheese are excellent sources of calcium, needed to build healthy bones and teeth, and to prevent osteoporosis, which can result in brittle bones and increased risk of fractures.

6. Tofu and other soy foods are thought to help reduce the risk of heart disease, ease menopausal symptoms and reduce the risk of cancer.

7. Whole grain bread is a good source of B vitamins. These vitamins help keep skin healthy by improving cellular metabolism. Whole grains are also rich in fiber which helps prevent constipation, and removes waste and toxins from the body.

*Tofu and other soy foods are thought to help reduce the risk of heart disease, ease menopausal symptoms and reduce the risk of cancer.*

8. Vegetable oil provides essential fatty acids for hormone production, is used to build and maintain cell walls and helps skin retain moisture.

9. Pineapple contains bromelain, an enzyme which may help the body restore collagen, repair damaged tissue and keep skin strong and supple.

10. Garlic is thought to boost the immune stystem, prevent heart disease and cancer, lower cholesterol and slow the ageing process.

# "Steam-Fried" Vegetables

Almost any combination of vegetables can be used for this dish. More or less garlic, ginger and low-sodium soy sauce can be used, to taste. Make up a batch of these veggies and keep them in the refrigerator for easy reheating in the microwave. Steam-frying is a great low-fat alternative to stir-frying.

**The Lowdown**
(per serving)

| | |
|---|---|
| calories | 55 |
| fat | 1 g |
| carbohydrates | 10 g |
| protein | 3 g |

| | | |
|---|---|---|
| | cooking spray | |
| ½ | Spanish onion, sliced | ½ |
| 2 | cloves garlic, minced | 2 |
| 1 tsp | minced fresh ginger | 5 mL |
| 1 | stalk broccoli, cut in florets and stems peeled and sliced | 1 |
| 1 | carrot, peeled and sliced | 1 |
| 1 | zucchini, sliced | 1 |
| ½ lb | mushrooms, sliced | 250 g |
| ½ each | green and red pepper, seeded and sliced in strips | ½ each |
| | ground pepper (to taste) | |
| 2 tbsp | low-sodium soy sauce | 25 mL |
| 1 tsp | sesame seed oil | 5 mL |

1. Cook onion, garlic and ginger in a small amount of water on medium-high heat in a non-stick pan or wok sprayed with cooking spray.
2. Add remaining vegetables, ½ cup / 125 mL water and low-sodium soy sauce. Season with fresh ground pepper. Steam-fry vegetables until broccoli turns a bright green color. Add small amounts of water as required.
3. Drizzle sesame seed oil over vegetables and cook for 1-2 minutes longer.

Makes 6 servings.

# Velvet Mashed Potatoes

So smooth and creamy, these are a dream. If you don't love garlic (or it doesn't love you), you can leave it out.

**The Lowdown**
For variety you can use a combination of white and sweet potatoes in this recipe.

| | | |
|---|---|---|
| 4 | Yukon gold potatoes, peeled and halved | 4 |
| 2-4 | cloves garlic | 2-4 |
| | water, to cover | |
| ½ tsp | black pepper | 2 mL |
| | salt (to taste) | |
| | chopped parsley | |

1. Place peeled potatoes and garlic in a small pot and add water to cover.
2. Cover pot and bring to a boil. Reduce heat and simmer until potatoes are soft.
3. Pour off water reserving ½ cup/125 mL cooking water.
4. Mash potatoes and garlic. Add black pepper, salt and small amounts of reserved cooking water until a creamy consistency is achieved.
5. Serve, sprinkled with chopped parsley.

Makes 4 servings.

# Oven French "Fries"

There's absolutely no reason to give up French fries when you can make these light and crispy oven "fries" at home.

| | | |
|---|---|---|
| | cooking spray | |
| 4 | large potatoes, unpeeled, washed and dried well, cut in strips | 4 |
| ½ tsp each | garlic powder, black pepper, paprika (or to taste) | 2 mL each |

**The Lowdown**
(per serving)

| | |
|---|---|
| calories | 151 |
| fat | 1 g |
| carbohydrates | 34 g |
| protein | 3 g |

1. Place potato strips on a baking sheet sprayed with cooking spray. Lightly spray potatoes with cooking spray.
2. Sprinkle potato strips with seasonings.
3. Bake in a 425°F/220°C oven for approximately 40 minutes, or until potatoes are tender inside and crisp on the outside.

Makes 4 servings.

# Baked Sweet Potato "Fries"

Sweet potatoes are nutrition dynamos, they're loaded with beta-carotene and packed with taste. These "fries" are wonderful with turkey, or as an anytime alternative to white potatoes or rice.

| | | |
|---|---|---|
| | cooking spray | |
| 4 | sweet potatoes, washed, unpeeled and cut into strips or wedges | 4 |
| | salt, black pepper (to taste) | |

1. Place sweet potato strips on a baking sheet sprayed with cooking spray. Lightly spray sweet potatoes with cooking spray.
2. Bake in a 425°F/220°C oven for approximately 40 minutes, or until potatoes are tender inside and crisp on the outside. Season to taste.

Makes 4 servings.

# Rosemary Roasted Taters

Rosemary is a fragrant herb that goes well with potatoes. Not only will you love the taste, you'll adore the aroma that fills your kitchen as these spuds bake in the oven.

|              | cooking spray                                       |        |
|--------------|-----------------------------------------------------|--------|
| 1½ lbs       | potatoes, washed, unpeeled, cut in wedges           | 750 g  |
| 1 tbsp       | dried rosemary                                      | 15 mL  |
| ½ tsp each   | garlic powder, black pepper (or to taste)           | 2 mL   |

1. Place potato wedges in a single layer on a non-stick baking sheet sprayed with cooking spray.
3. Lightly spray potato wedges with cooking spray. Sprinkle with seasonings.
2. Bake in a 425°F/220°C oven for 40 minutes or until potatoes are cooked and crispy.

Makes 6 servings.

**The Lowdown**
**(per serving)**

| calories      | 129  |
|---------------|------|
| fat           | 0 g  |
| carbohydrates | 29 g |
| protein       | 3 g  |

**Highlight**

You can oven roast other vegetables like sweet potatoes, carrots, squash, onions and parsnips, alone or in combination using this method. Make a large batch that you can keep in the refrigerator and reheat as needed.

# Cranapple Red Cabbage

**The Lowdown**
(per serving)

| | |
|---|---|
| calories | 55 |
| fat | 0 g |
| carbohydrates | 14 g |
| protein | 1 g |

Serve this lovely ruby-colored side-dish hot or cold with turkey or chicken. On festive occasions, your family and guests will appreciate this light addition to balance out traditional higher fat fare.

| | | |
|---|---|---|
| 1 lb | red cabbage, shredded | 500 g |
| 1 cup | water | 250 mL |
| ½ cup | canned cranberry sauce (whole berry) | 125 mL |
| 1 | apple, cored, peeled, thinly sliced | 1 |
| ½ cup | orange juice | 125 mL |
| ½ tsp | grated orange rind (optional) | 2 mL |
| ½ tsp | cinnamon | 2 mL |
| ½ tsp | nutmeg | 2 mL |
| ½ tsp each | salt, black pepper (or to taste) | 2 mL each |

1. Place red cabbage in a pot with 1 cup/250 mL of water. Bring to a boil, reduce heat and cook covered on low heat for a few minutes until the cabbage starts to wilt.
2. Add sliced apples, orange juice, cranberry sauce and seasonings. Stir mixture, cover and simmer over low heat until cabbage and apples are soft, about 30 minutes.

Makes 8 servings.

# CHAPTER 15

# *Protein Power*

C ONTRARY TO WHAT YOU MIGHT THNK, you don't have to eat skinless chicken breasts and water-packed tuna every day of the week to achieve your healthy eating and weight goals. In fact, limiting your choices will only put you at risk of developing a major case of boredom. We all know how dangerous that can be when you're trying to eat in a healthy way.

Let's review the Fab Four when it comes to eating poultry, meat and fish, so you'll recall how you can eat them all.

The first is to eat these foods lean and well-trimmed. Ask your butcher for guidance if you're not sure which are the leanest cuts. Cut away all visible fat before cooking and eating. Don't forget to remove poultry skin and skip the wings, which are loaded with fat.

The second is to use a low-fat cooking method like roasting on a rack, broiling, steaming, poaching, baking, microwaving or grilling. Avoid frying. Whether it's pan frying or deep frying, both add plenty of fat. Instead, "steam-fry" using broth or water in the pan, or stir-fry with a bit of water, low-sodium soy sauce and a touch of oil.

The third is to aim for a three-ounce (100 g) portion of cooked protein. That's about four ounces (125 g) raw . You can

*Limiting your choices will only put you at risk of developing a major case of boredom.*

eyeball your portion. Or you can buy a food scale. It's a very useful and inexpensive tool to have in your kitchen.

A three-ounce (100 g) portion is about the size of a deck of cards or the palm of your hand. If this sounds skimpy to you, remember two of these is probably all your body needs along with the protein in other foods for your protein requirements.

A great way to stick to the recommended serving size is to enjoy mixed dishes where the meat or poultry is an ingredient rather than the main event. For example, instead of a roast of beef, enjoy a few meatballs with tomato sauce and rice. Grilled chicken strips in a spicy fajita is preferable to a half-chicken entrée. A veal stew packed with veggies is a lighter choice than a veal chop. Soon, it will become second nature for you to plan meals this way.

The last Fab Four is variety, the bottom line of healthy eating. We need fifty nutrients or more each day for good health. By enjoying a wide variety of foods you have the best chance of getting them all. A variety of poultry, meat, fish and alternatives lets you have them all without feeling bored or deprived.

> *A variety of poultry, meat, fish and alternatives lets you have them all without feeling bored or deprived.*

## Meat of the Matter

1. Pre-packaged ground chicken and turkey are good alternatives for ground beef, as long as the skin hasn't been ground in too. You can have the butcher grind skinless chicken or turkey for you. Or you can use one of the defatting methods suggested in the recipes.

2. When handling raw poultry, keep it away from other foods which will be served raw, like salads and fruit. Wash your hands, utensils and cutting boards very well after handling.

3. Always thoroughly cook chicken. Never eat it pink or undercooked.

4. The leanest cuts of beef include round, sirloin and tenderloin.

5. When using meat as an ingredient in a recipe, refrigerate after cooking. Remove the hardened fat before reheating and serving.

6. After browning ground meats, pour off the liquid fat, and rinse meat with warm water to wash away traces of fat.

7. Serve your burgers and meatloaf well done. Never eat undercooked ground meat, which can contain very harmful bacteria.

8. The amount of fat in fish varies. The good news is that fatty fish contains heart-healthy omega-3 fatty acids. Balance your intake of higher-fat fish like salmon, swordfish and herring with lower fat choices such as sole, haddock, halibut and most seafood.

9. When ordering fish in a restaurant, ask for your fish broiled or grilled without fat. If you just ask for no butter, they may use oil and plenty of it.

10. Take care not to overcook fish. Bake fish in a hot oven 425°F/220°C for 10 minutes per inch/2.5 cm thickness of fresh fish, 20 minutes per inch/2.5 cm thickness if it's frozen.

11. Fish is done when it flakes easily with a fork and is opaque (no longer translucent).

*After browning ground meats, pour off the liquid fat, and rinse meat with warm water to wash away traces of fat.*

# Protein Power Recipes

# Fasta Pasta with Meat Sauce

This recipe is so quick and easy to make, you'll get dinner ready in record time. Serve with a salad to start and fresh fruit for dessert. Delicioso!

| | | |
|---|---|---|
| 1 lb | extra-lean ground beef | 500 g |
| 3 cups | pasta sauce (meatless) | 750 mL |
| 8 oz | dry pasta | 250 g |

1. In a large non-stick saucepan, brown ground meat on medium heat until no longer pink. Pour off fat. Rinse meat with tap water. Return pan with meat to stove.
2. Stir in pasta sauce and bring to a boil. Reduce heat and simmer covered on low heat for about 30 minutes.
3. In a large pot of boiling water, cook pasta until tender but firm, al dente.
4. Drain pasta. To serve, toss pasta with sauce.

Makes 6 servings.

### The Lowdown
(per serving )

| | |
|---|---|
| calories | 359 |
| fat | 10 g |
| carbohydrate | 43 g |
| protein | 22 g |

### Highlight
You can use ground veal, chicken or turkey in place of the beef.

# Soy Good Lasagna

This light yet hearty main dish combines the best of all worlds—iron-rich lean ground beef, soy protein-packed tofu cheese and anti-oxidant powered mixed vegetables. And it tastes great too!

### The Lowdown
(per serving)

| | |
|---|---|
| calories | 299 |
| fat | 8 g |
| carbohydrate | 32 g |
| protein | 24 g |

### Highlight

To go completely vegetarian and to increase the soy protein, substitute soy ground "beef" for the extra-lean ground beef.

| | | |
|---|---|---|
| 1 lb | extra-lean ground beef | 500 g |
| 1 | onion, chopped | 1 |
| 1-2 | garlic cloves, minced | 1-2 |
| 1 tsp | Italian seasonings | 5 mL |
| 4 cups | pasta sauce (meatless) | 1 L |
| 9 | oven-ready lasagna noodles | 9 |
| 8 oz | fat-free tofu cheese (Mozzarella flavor) | 250 g |
| 2 cups | frozen Italian vegetables | 500 mL |

1. In a non-stick pot, brown ground beef on medium heat until no longer pink. Pour off fat, rinse meat with water. Return pot with meat to stove.
2. Add chopped onion, garlic, Italian seasonings and 1 cup/250 mL pasta sauce. Stir to combine.
3. Simmer meat mixture on medium heat uncovered for 10 minutes. Set aside.
4. To assemble lasagna, spread 1 cup/250 mL pasta sauce on bottom of lasagna pan.
5. Cover with 3 lasagna noodles.
6. Spread meat mixture over noodles. Cover with 3 lasagna noodles.
7. Spread noodles with 1 cup/250 mL pasta sauce. Top with shredded tofu cheese. Spread frozen vegetables over tofu cheese.
8. Cover with last 3 noodles. Spread remaining sauce over noodles.
9. Bake covered in a 375°F/190°C oven for 1½ hours.
10. Remove lasagna from oven and allow to rest for 15 minutes before cutting.

Makes 8 servings.

# Mighty Good Meatballs

These meatballs are always a hit. You can reduce the amount of sugar or sweetener if you like them less sweet. Serve over rice or noodles with steamed veggies and fresh fruit for dessert.

| | | |
|---|---|---|
| 1 lb | extra-lean ground beef | 500 g |
| 4 | egg whites or ½ cup/125 mL egg whites in a carton, lightly beaten | 4 |
| ½ cup | bread or cracker crumbs, or matzo meal | 125 mL |
| ½ tsp | garlic powder | 2 mL |
| ½ tsp | black pepper | 2 mL |
| ½ tsp | Worcestershire sauce | 2 mL |
| ½ tsp | salt (or to taste) | 2 mL |
| 1 | 28 oz / 796 mL can crushed tomatoes | 1 |
| 2 tbsp | ketchup | 25 mL |
| ¼ cup | white sugar or equivalent sweetener | 50 mL |
| 2 tbsp | balsamic vinegar or lemon juice black pepper (to taste) | 25 mL |

**The Lowdown**
(per serving)

| | |
|---|---|
| calories | 276 |
| fat | 10 g |
| carbohydrate | 27 g |
| protein | 20 g |

**Highlight**

You can use ground veal, chicken or turkey in place of the beef.

1. Combine first seven ingredients.
2. Fill a large non-stick pot half full with water. Bring water to a boil.
3. With wet hands form meatballs and gently place meatballs in water.
4. Simmer meatballs over medium-high heat. Skim off any foam that forms.
5. When meatballs are cooked and no longer pink, remove meatballs from water with a slotted spoon. Pour off the water, rinse out pot and place meatballs back into the pot.
5. In a bowl combine crushed tomatoes, ketchup, sugar and balsamic vinegar and pour over meatballs. Season with fresh ground pepper, if desired.
6. Bring to a boil. Cover and simmer gently for 1 hour.

Makes 6 servings.

# Fit'n Trim Meat Loaf

This meat loaf is a popular "light" choice served at the Club restaurant at The Fitness Institute. It's a wonderful hot entrée with garlicky mashed potatoes and steamed broccoli. You can also enjoy it cold on a sandwich slathered with Dijon mustard.

| | | |
|---|---|---|
| 1 lb | extra-lean ground beef | 500 g |
| 4 | egg whites or ½ cup / 125 mL egg whites in a carton, lightly beaten | 4 |
| ½ cup | bread or cracker crumbs, or matzo meal | 125 mL |
| ½ tsp | garlic powder | 2 mL |
| ½ tsp | black pepper | 2 mL |
| 1 tbsp | ketchup | 15 mL |
| ½ tsp | salt (or to taste) | 2 mL |
| | cooking spray | |
| | paprika | |

1. Combine first seven ingredients well.
2. Spray a small loaf pan with cooking spray.
3. Turn meat mixture into loaf pan. Sprinkle the top with paprika.
4. Bake in a 350°F/180C oven for about 1 hour or until meat loaf is thoroughly cooked.
5. To serve, remove meat loaf from pan and cut into slices.

Makes 6 servings.

# Ship-Shape Shepherd's Pie

This light version of a family favorite is satisfying and very easy to make. Serve with a mixed salad and fresh fruit for dessert.

| | | |
|---|---|---|
| 1 lb | extra-lean ground beef | 500 g |
| 1 | onion, chopped | 1 |
| ½ cup | crushed tomatoes | 125 mL |
| ½ cup | water | 125 mL |
| 2 tbsp | ketchup | 25 mL |
| 1 tsp | mustard (yellow or Dijon) | 5 mL |
| 1 tsp | Worcestershire sauce | 5 mL |
| ½ tsp | black pepper | 2 mL |
| | salt (to taste) | |
| 2 cups | frozen California vegetables | 500 mL |
| ½ cup | frozen green peas | 125 mL |
| ½ cup | frozen corn niblets | 125 mL |
| 4 | potatoes, peeled, cooked and mashed | 4 |
| ¼ tsp | paprika | 1 mL |

**The Lowdown**
(per serving halibut)

| | |
|---|---|
| calories | 257 |
| fat | 9 g |
| carbohydrate | 26 g |
| protein | 18 g |

**Highlight**

You can use ground veal, chicken or turkey in place of the beef.

1. Brown ground meat in a non-stick pot. Pour off fat. Rinse meat with warm water.
2. Return pot with meat to stove. Add chopped onion to meat and continue to cook until onion is softened.
3. Add remaining ingredients except potatoes. Bring to a boil and simmer uncovered for 20 minutes.
4. Spoon meat and vegetable mixture into an 8-inch/2 L square baking dish. Top with mashed potatoes and smooth evenly over meat mixture. Sprinkle with paprika.
5. Bake in a 350°F/180°C oven for 20 minutes or until potatoes are golden brown.

Makes 6 servings.

# Heart-Smart Veal Stew

Enjoy this stew to your healthy heart's content. Make it a day ahead if possible, so it can be refrigerated and the hardened fat can be removed before reheating.

**The Lowdown**
(per serving)

| | |
|---|---|
| calories | 229 |
| fat | 4 g |
| carbohydrate | 24 g |
| protein | 24 g |

| | | |
|---|---|---|
| 1 lb | stewing veal, trimmed and cubed | 500 g |
| 2 tbsp | flour | 25 mL |
| ½ tsp each | garlic powder, pepper, paprika | 2 mL each |
| | cooking spray | |
| 4 cups | defatted chicken broth | 1 L |
| | few dashes Worcestershire sauce | |
| 1 | bay leaf | 1 |
| 4 | potatoes, peeled and cubed | 4 |
| 2 | carrots, peeled and sliced | 2 |
| 1 | celery stalk, sliced | 1 |
| 1 | onion, diced | 1 |
| 2 tbsp | chopped parsley | 25 mL |
| ½ cup | frozen peas | 125 mL |
| ½ cup | frozen corn niblets | 125 mL |
| | salt, pepper (to taste) | |

1. Season veal cubes lightly with garlic powder, pepper and paprika. Dredge veal with flour. Shake off excess.
2. On medium-high heat, lightly brown veal cubes in a large non-stick soup pot sprayed with cooking spray.
3. Add chicken broth, bay leaf and a few dashes Worcestershire sauce. Cover pot and simmer gently for 1 hour.
4. Add vegetables and continue cooking for about ½ hour or until vegetables are tender. Add frozen peas and corn during last 10 minutes of cooking. Season with salt and pepper, to taste.
5. To serve, remove bay leaf and ladle into soup bowls.

Makes 6 servings.

# Fabulous Fajitas

These are easy to make and lots of fun to eat. You may want to spice these fajitas with hot pepper sauce or salsa. Go ahead. Both are fat-free.

| | | |
|---|---|---|
| 4 | chicken breasts, boneless and skinless, cut in strips seasoned with black pepper, garlic powder, chili powder, paprika (to taste) | 4 |
| 4 | medium-size flour tortillas | 4 |
| 1 cup | shredded lettuce | 250 mL |
| 1 | large tomato, diced | 1 |
| 2 | green onions, sliced | 2 |
| ½ cup | salsa | 125 mL |
| ½ cup | plain fat-free yogurt | 125 mL |
| 2 oz | low-fat cheddar cheese, shredded | 50 g |

1. On a serving plate, arrange lettuce, tomato and green onions.
2. On a second serving plate, place salsa, yogurt and shredded cheese.
3. Grill, broil or BBQ seasoned chicken strips. Set aside and keep warm.
5. Warm tortillas for a few seconds in the microwave, and cover with a napkin.

**To assemble:**

1. Spread tortilla with 2 tbsp / 25 mL each salsa and yogurt. Place a few chicken strips, shredded lettuce, tomato and green onions in center of tortilla. Sprinkle with low-fat cheddar cheese.
2. Roll up fajita and enjoy.

Makes 4 fajitas.

# Chicken Fingers

Serve these crispy, tender chicken fingers plain or with honey mustard, plum sauce or ketchup for dipping. Partially freezing the chicken breasts makes them very easy to slice.

| **The Lowdown** (per serving) | |
|---|---|
| calories | 238 |
| fat | 3 g |
| carbohydrate | 21 g |
| protein | 30 g |

| | | |
|---|---|---|
| 1 lb | skinless, boneless chicken breasts | 500 g |
| ½ tsp | seasoned salt | 2 mL |
| 4 | egg whites or ½ cup/125 mL egg whites in a carton, lightly beaten | 4 |
| 1 cup | cornflake crumbs | 250 mL |
| | cooking spray | |

1. Slice chicken breasts across the grain into ½"/1 cm wide strips.
2. Sprinkle chicken strips with seasoned salt.
3. Place cornflake crumbs on a plate.
4. Pour egg whites into a shallow bowl.
5. Dip chicken strips into lightly beaten egg whites.
6. Roll chicken strips in crumbs to coat.
7. Place coated chicken strips in a single layer on a non-stick baking sheet sprayed with cooking spray. Spray chicken strips lightly with cooking spray before baking.
8. Bake in a 375°F/190°C oven for 30 minutes or until chicken strips are cooked and no longer pink inside.

Makes 4 servings.

# Lean-ing Tower Pasta with Chicken

This dish will make you think of the famous tower in Pisa because it's so "lean".

| | | |
|---|---|---|
| | cooking spray | |
| 4 | skinless boneless chicken breasts cut in strips | 4 |
| 1 tsp | minced garlic | 5 mL |
| | black pepper (to taste) | |
| 2 cups | frozen Italian vegetables (broccoli, carrots, cauliflower, green beans) | 500 mL |
| 3 cups | pasta sauce (meatless) | 750 mL |
| 2 tbsp | chopped basil or 1 tsp/5 mL dried | 25 mL |
| 8 oz | rotini or penne pasta, uncooked | 250 g |

1. Season chicken strips with black papper. In a non-stick pot sprayed with cooking spray, cook the chicken strips and garlic in a little water until chicken is no longer pink.
2. Add pasta sauce, basil and frozen vegetables. Cover pot and simmer on low heat for 20 minutes.
3. In the meantime, bring a large pot of water to a boil. Cook pasta until tender but firm. Drain pasta.
4. To serve, place 1 cup/250 mL pasta on plate. Spoon chicken, vegetables and sauce on top.

Makes 6 servings.

# Just Peachy Chicken Breasts

The flavor of peaches goes wonderfully well with chicken. Serve over couscous with a medley of steamed veggies.

| | | |
|---|---|---|
| | cooking spray | |
| 4 | skinless boneless chicken breasts | 4 |
| 1 tsp | minced garlic | 5 mL |
| | black pepper (to taste) | |
| 4 tbsp | peach or apricot fruit spread | 50 mL |
| 4 tbsp | low-sodium soy sauce | 50 mL |

1. Combine minced garlic, fruit spread, soy sauce and pepper in a glass baking dish.
2. Add chicken breasts, turn to coat, cover and refrigerate for at least 2 hours or overnight. Turn chicken pieces occasionally, if possible.
3. Bake uncovered in a 350°F / 180°C oven for about 30-40 minutes, basting occasionally until chicken is thoroughly cooked and browned.

Makes 4 servings.

# Aloha Chicken

You'll soon be thinking about grass skirts and palm trees swaying on the beach at Waikiki when you bite into this succulent chicken dish.

| | | |
|---|---|---|
| 1 cup | tomato juice | 250 mL |
| 2 tbsp | low-sodium soy sauce | 25 mL |
| 2 tbsp | seasoned rice vinegar | 25 mL |
| 1 | 19 oz / 540 mL can sliced pineapple in its own juice | 1 |
| 1 tsp | minced garlic | 5 mL |
| ¼ tsp | black pepper | 1 mL |
| 4 | skinless chicken breasts | 4 |
| 1 tsp | sesame seeds | 5 mL |

**The Lowdown**
(per serving)

| | |
|---|---|
| calories | 253 |
| fat | 3 g |
| carbohydrate | 29 g |
| protein | 27 g |

1. To make marinade, combine tomato juice, soy sauce, vinegar, juice from pineapple, garlic and black pepper in a large glass baking dish.
2. Add chicken breasts, turn to coat, cover and marinate in refrigerator for at least 2 hours or overnight.
3. When ready to bake, top chicken breasts with pineapple slices and sprinkle with sesame seeds. If you find there is too much liquid, pour off some before baking.
4. Bake in a 350°F / 180°C oven uncovered for 1 hour or until chicken is thoroughly cooked and no longer pink inside. If using boneless breasts, the cooking time will be shorter.

Makes 4 servings.

# Dip'n Bake Chicken

The low-calorie salad dressing adds flavor to the chicken and makes it tender and juicy. The cornflake crumbs give the chicken a golden brown color without frying.

| | | |
|---|---|---|
| 4 | skinless chicken breasts | 4 |
| ½ cup | low-calorie or fat-free Italian or Catalina salad dressing | 125 mL |
| 1 cup | cornflake crumbs | 250 mL |
| | cooking spray | |

1. Marinate chicken breasts in low-calorie salad dressing in the refrigerator for at least 2 hours or overnight.
2. Pour cornflake crumbs onto a plate. Remove each chicken breast from marinade, shake off excess and dip into crumbs to coat thoroughly.
3. Place coated chicken breasts in a shallow baking pan sprayed with cooking spray.
5. Bake in a 350°F/180°C oven for 1 hour or until chicken is thoroughly cooked and crispy.

Makes 4 servings.

## The Lowdown
(per serving)

| | |
|---|---|
| calories | 236 |
| fat | 4 g |
| carbohydrate | 22 g |
| protein | 27 g |

## Highlight

If using boneless chicken breasts, baking time will be shorter. Be careful not to overcook.

Legs and thighs can be used in this recipe. The calorie and fat content will be somewhat higher.

# Citrus Marinade for Poultry

Try this marinade the next time you grill chicken. Studies show that marinating meats and poultry before BBQing decreases the risk of potentially harmful chemicals being formed and deposited on your food. Good tasting and good for you too—the perfect combination.

| | | |
|---|---|---|
| 2 tbsp | lime juice | 25 mL |
| ¼ cup | orange juice | 50 mL |
| 2 tbsp | low-sodium soy sauce | 25 mL |
| 1-2 | cloves garlic, minced | 1-2 |
| ½ tsp | minced ginger (or to taste) | 2 mL |
| ½ tsp | cumin (or to taste) | 2 mL |

1. Combine marinade ingredients.
2. Pour over skinless chicken pieces, cover and let stand in refrigerator for 1 hour or overnight.
3. Discard marinade and grill chicken until thoroughly cooked.

Makes ½ cup / 125 mL marinade.

**The Lowdown**
(per 1 tbsp / 15 mL)

| | |
|---|---|
| calories | 6 |
| fat | 0 g |
| carbohydrate | 2 g |
| protein | 0 g |

# Heart and Sole

**The Lowdown**
(per serving)

| | |
|---|---|
| calories | 166 |
| fat | 2 g |
| carbohydrate | 11 g |
| protein | 25 g |

You can make your own tartar sauce for this light and easy fish dish by combining ¼ cup/50 mL ultra-light or fat-free mayonnaise with a teaspoon or two of relish. Serve with oven "fries" and steamed veggies. Fish and chips never tasted so good!

| | cooking spray | |
|---|---|---|
| 1 lb | filet of sole | 500 g |
| ½ tsp each | garlic powder, salt, black pepper, paprika (or to taste) | 2 mL each |
| ½ cup | cornflake crumbs | 125 mL |
| 4 | egg whites or ½ cup/125 mL egg whites in a carton, lightly beaten | 4 |
| 1 | lemon, quartered (for garnish) | 1 |

1. Spray non-stick baking sheet with cooking spray.
2. Lightly season sole with garlic powder, salt, black pepper and paprika.
3. Spread cornflake crumbs on a plate. Pour egg whites into a shallow bowl.
4. Dip sole filets in egg whites and then roll in cornflake crumbs to coat.
5. Place on non-stick baking sheet sprayed cooking spray. Lightly spray tops of fish.
6. Bake in a 425°F/220°C oven for 10 minutes per inch /2.5 cm thickness of fish or until fish is opaque and flakes easily with a fork.
7. Serve immediately, garnished with a lemon quarter.

Makes 4 servings.

# Ginger Fish Fillets

These fish fillets can be baked in the oven or grilled on the BBQ. The exotic flavors marry well with even the most distinctive tasting fish like salmon or swordfish.

| | | |
|---|---|---|
| 2 tbsp | puréed fresh ginger | 25 mL |
| 1 tsp | Dijon mustard | 5 mL |
| 2 tsp | balsamic vinegar | 10 mL |
| | black pepper (to taste) | |
| 1 tsp | minced garlic | 5 mL |
| 1 tbsp | chopped cilantro or parsley | 15 mL |
| | cooking spray | |
| 1 lb | fish fillets (halibut, tuna, haddock, salmon, or swordfish) | 500 g |

1. In a small bowl combine ginger, mustard, balsamic vinegar, black pepper, garlic and cilantro.
2. Place fish fillets in a baking dish sprayed with cooking spray.
3. Spread ginger mixture on fish to coat evenly.
4. Bake in a 425°F/220°C oven for 10 minutes per inch/2.5 cm thickness of fish or until fish is opaque and flakes easily with a fork.

Makes 4 servings.

## The Lowdown
**(per serving halibut)**

| | |
|---|---|
| calories | 136 |
| fat | 3 g |
| carbohydrate | 2 g |
| protein | 24 g |

## Highlight

**For tapenade fish fillets:**

Instead of ginger mixture, top fish fillets with a mixture of 2 tbsp/25 mL chopped black olives, 1 diced tomato, 2 tsp/5 mL chopped capers, 2 tbsp/25 mL chopped fresh basil, black pepper and garlic.

**For Mexican fish fillets:**

Top fish fillets with salsa instead of ginger mixture.

The fat and calorie content will vary depending on the topping and fish used.

# Mediterranean Fish Stew

You can use shrimp, scallops or mussels in place of some or all of the fish in this flavorful recipe. Serve with crusty Italian bread for dipping. You won't want to miss one drop of the delicious tomato broth.

| | | |
|---|---|---|
| 1 tsp | olive oil | 5 mL |
| 2 | cloves garlic, minced | 2 |
| 2 tbsp | chopped parsley | 25 mL |
| 1 tsp | cumin | 5 mL |
| 1 tsp | paprika | 5 mL |
| ¼ tsp | hot pepper flakes or hot sauce | 1 mL |
| 1 | 28 oz / 796 mL can tomatoes, broken in pieces | 1 |
| | juice of 1 lemon | |
| 1 tbsp | sugar (or equivalent sweetener) | 15 mL |
| 1 lb | fish fillets (haddock, halibut red snapper, or tilapia) | 500 g |
| 4 | sprigs parsley or cilantro | 4 |

1. Heat olive oil in large nonstick saucepan, add garlic and cook on medium heat until golden.
2. Add chopped parsley, cumin, paprika and hot pepper flakes. Cook for 1 minute more.
3. Add canned tomatoes, bring to a boil, reduce heat and simmer covered for 10 minutes.
4. Add lemon juice and sugar.
5. Place fish fillets on tomato mixture. Top each fish fillet with 1 sprig parsley.
6. Cover and cook on low heat for about 30 minutes, or until fish is cooked and flakes easily with a fork.

Makes 4 servings.

# Terrific Tuna

At the deli counter, go for a turkey, sliced chicken or lean meat sandwich piled high with veggies on whole grain bread. Save the tuna for the weekend when you can make this low-fat version at home.

| | | |
|---|---|---|
| 1 | 6 oz / 170 g can water-packed tuna, drained | 1 |
| 2 tbsp | ultra-light or fat-free mayonnaise | 25 mL |
| ¼ tsp | black pepper | 1 mL |
| 1 tsp | chopped parsley or dill (optional) | 5 mL |

1. Place all ingredients in a food processor fitted with the steel knife.
2. Process with a few on-off pulses until tuna is light and fluffy. Be careful not to over-process.

Makes 3 servings.

## The Lowdown
**(per serving)**

| | |
|---|---|
| calories | 63 |
| fat | 1 g |
| carbohydrate | 2 g |
| protein | 11 g |

## Highlight

You can add veggies to your Terrific Tuna like chopped celery, green onion, red or green pepper, if you wish.

This recipe works well with canned salmon or hard-boiled eggs, but the calorie and fat content will be higher. To reduce the fat content of chopped egg, use one whole egg and several egg whites.

# Svelte Tuna Melt

When you're in the mood for a light meal with a minimum of fuss and bother, try this open-face sandwich teamed with a steaming bowl of vegetable soup.

**The Lowdown**
(per serving)

| | |
|---|---|
| calories | 189 |
| fat | 5 g |
| carbohydrate | 17 g |
| protein | 18 g |

| | cooking spray | |
|---|---|---|
| 1 slice | whole wheat or rye bread | 1 slice |
| 1 serving | Terrific Tuna | 1 serving |
| ½ oz | part-skim Mozzarella cheese | 15 g |

1. Place slice of bread on a baking sheet sprayed with cooking spray. Spread bread with Terrific Tuna. Sprinkle with part-skim Mozzarella cheese.
2. Place under the broiler until bread is toasted and cheese is melted.

Makes 1 serving.

## CHAPTER 16

# Be My Guest

YOU NO LONGER HAVE TO WORRY that special occasion eating will sabotage your healthy eating and weight goals. Don't burden yourself with unnecessary concern. Special occasions are a wonderful time to be with family and friends, so relax and enjoy yourself. You can have a good time and see the light too.

We all know that traditional holiday recipes tend to be high in fat and calories. Have you ever wondered why? My view is that when these recipes were first created, it was a time when people needed many more calories than we do today. These days, machines do most of the physical work for us, so we can get by on far fewer calories. Yet we still prepare and eat many of the same high-calorie recipes, particularly on special occasions.

In the past, food wasn't as plentiful and readily available as it is now. Special occasion eating took place only a few times a year. Being so infrequent, it was a fine opportunity to indulge in an abundance of higher fat foods. In time, the groaning board became a symbol of bounty, happiness and good fortune. No wonder today we think that no holiday has been properly celebrated until we're all groaning from how

> *Special occasions are a wonderful time to be with family and friends, so relax and enjoy yourself. You can have a good time and see the light too.*

much we've eaten. Regardless of how much we complain, the tradition continues.

In addition, for many in North America, happily, special occasion eating can take place almost every day. Birthday or anniversary celebrations, dinner parties, Superbowl or Grey Cup Sundays, Christmas, Chanukah, New Year's, Passover, Easter and other traditional holidays are always on the horizon. The fat and calories can really add up if you're not careful. The only way to survive and enjoy these special occasions is to see the light.

When you're the host, show your guests how much you really care by treating them to lighter fare. My clients and I do this all the time. And no one feels deprived if the spirit of the occasion remains intact.

Party dips can be made with fat-free sour cream or low-fat cottage cheese, baked bagel and pita crisps replace deep-fried potato and corn chips. Egg whites can be used whenever possible in cooking and baking instead of whole eggs. Foods can be "fried" in non-stick pans sprayed with cooking spray. It's all about using a lighter touch.

*Lighten up your own recipes by using many of the cooking techniques you've been learning along the way.*

This chapter contains a potpourri of lighter dishes for special occasions. Lighten up your own recipes by using many of the cooking techniques you've been learning along the way. And be sure to serve any one of the recipes in this book to your guests with confidence and pride. You don't have to let them know that the great tasting food you're serving is good for them too, until after they start asking for seconds.

## Special Occasion Tips

1. Whip low-fat cottage cheese in the food processor as a base for creamy dips.

2. Plain or seasoned baked bagel and pita crisps are a great way to use up leftover bagels and pita.

3. Equal parts of fruit juice and non-cola, sugar-free soft drinks make refreshing non-alcoholic spritzers. Serve over ice garnished with lemon or lime.

4. Be sure to serve plenty of vegetable side-dishes to balance higher fat and calorie choices.

5. Whatever dessert is being served, always include fresh fruit as an alternative or as a complement.

*Whatever dessert is being served, always include fresh fruit as an alternative or as a complement.*

# Special Occasion Recipes

# Fit To Be Tried Spinach Dip

We used to make this dip with one cup each regular mayonnaise and sour cream. And we thought it was a healthy choice because we ate it with veggies.

| | | |
|---|---|---|
| 1 cup | 1% cottage cheese | 250 mL |
| 2 tbsp | lemon juice | 25 mL |
| 1 cup | fat-free sour cream | 250 mL |
| 1 | 10 oz / 300 g package frozen chopped spinach, thawed and drained of excess water | 1 |
| 1 cup | sliced water chestnuts | 250 mL |
| 2 | cloves garlic, sliced | 2 |
| 2 | green onions, sliced | 2 |
| 1 tsp | salt (or to taste) | 5 mL |
| 2 tbsp | fresh parsley, chopped | 25 mL |
| ½ tsp | black pepper (or to taste) | 2 mL |
| | round pumpernickel bread | |
| | assorted raw veggies (cucumber slices, carrot sticks, red and green pepper rings, mushroom caps, celery sticks) | |

1. In food processor fitted with the steel blade, whip cottage cheese with lemon juice until smooth.
2. Add sour cream, spinach, water chestnuts, green onions, garlic, parsley, salt and black pepper. Process until smooth.
3. Transfer to a bowl, cover and refrigerate until ready to serve.
4. To serve, cut off top of pumpernickel bread and hollow out center. Cut bread from center into large cubes.
5. Place hollowed out bread on a round platter. Fill bread with dip. Garnish platter with bread cubes and assorted raw veggies.

Makes 4 cups / 1 L dip.

## The Lowdown
(per 1 tbsp/15 mL dip)

| | |
|---|---|
| calories | 7 |
| fat | 0 g |
| carbohydrate | 1 g |
| protein | 1 g |

## Highlight

If you're feeling really extravagant, replace the spinach and water chestnuts with 2 oz/50 g smoked salmon. Serve in the hollowed out pumpernickel bread and dot the surface of the dip with a few teaspoons of red or black caviar. Garnish the platter with the bread cubes and raw veggies. Most impressive!

# Bagel Crisps

This is a great way to recycle leftover bagels. These crisps are terrific for dipping, are wonderful with a bowl of soup and can be eaten just like melba toast.

| | | |
|---|---|---|
| 2 | 3 oz/100 g bagels | 2 |
| | cooking spray | |
| ½ tsp each | black pepper, garlic powder and rosemary | 2 mL each |

1. To slice bagel, place it on cutting board. With a sharp knife, carefully cut each bagel into thin slices, vertically instead of horizontally.
2. Place bagel slices on a cookie sheet sprayed with cooking spray.
3. Spray bagel slices lightly with cooking spray. Sprinkle with seasonings.
4. Bake in a 425°F/220°C oven for 8-10 minutes, or until toasted and crispy. Watch them carefully to make sure they don't burn.

Makes 6 servings.

## The Lowdown
(per 1oz/30 g serving)

| | |
|---|---|
| calories | 82 |
| fat | 1 g |
| carbohydrate | 15 g |
| protein | 3 g |

## Highlight

You can do the same with pita bread. Cut each pita into 8 wedges and follow this method.

# Greyhound Spritzer

A popular drink made with grapefruit juice is called the Greyhound. Try one of these instead of a high-cal cocktail.

| ½ cup | grapefruit juice | 125 mL |
| ½ cup | sugar-free, non-cola soft drink | 125 mL |
| | fresh lime | |
| | ice cubes | |

**The Lowdown**
(per spritzer)

| | |
|---|---|
| calories | 47 |
| fat | 0 g |
| carbohydrate | 11 g |
| protein | 1 g |

1. Place ice cubes in a highball glass. Pour grapefruit juice over ice cubes.
2. Fill glass with a sugar-free, non-cola soft drink. Garnish with a squeeze of fresh lime.

Makes 1 spritzer.

# It's My Party Punch

You won't feel like "crying" when you taste this refreshing drink. This version has a new "Twist". It's minus much of the sugar and many of the calories in regular punch.

| 4 cups | sugar-free, non-cola soft drink | 1 L |
| 4 cups | cranberry juice cocktail | 1 L |
| 1 | 6 oz / 176 mL canned frozen orange juice concentrate | 1 |
| 1½ cups | ice cubes | 375 mL |
| | orange, lemon and lime slices (for garnish) | |

**The Lowdown**
(per ½ cup/125 mL)

| | |
|---|---|
| calories | 46 |
| fat | 0 g |
| carbohydrate | 11 g |
| protein | 0 g |

1. Combine ingredients in a large punch bowl.
2. Stir well and add ice cubes just before serving.
3. Garnish with thin slices of orange, lemon and lime.

Makes 10 cups.

# Monday Night Munch Mix

**The Lowdown**
**(per ½ cup/125 mL)**

| | |
|---|---|
| calories | 67 |
| fat | 3 g |
| carbohydrate | 9 g |
| protein | 2 g |

Serve this mix to your pals when they come over to watch the game. Or pack one-cup/250 mL servings in sandwich bags as lunch-box treats. Store leftover mix in an air-tight container.

| | | |
|---|---|---|
| 1 cup | crispy rice cereal | 250 mL |
| 1 cup | shredded wheat cereal squares | 250 mL |
| 1½ cups | toasted oat cereal | 375 mL |
| 1 cup | pretzels (small size) | 250 mL |
| 3 cups | air-popped popcorn | 750 mL |
| ½ cup | dry-roasted peanuts | 125 mL |

1. Combine ingredients in a large bowl.

Makes 8 cups/2 L munch mix.

# Grilled Veggie Gourmet Pizza

I first served these gourmet pizzas at a family get-together. The flour tortillas make thin and crispy crusts and come in a variety of flavors.

| | | |
|---|---|---|
| | olive oil flavored cooking spray | |
| ½ each | red, yellow and green peppers, seeded and cut in strips | ½ each |
| 2 | zucchinis, sliced in rounds | 2 |
| 4 | portobello mushroom caps | 4 |
| | dried rosemary, black pepper (to taste) | |
| 8 | medium flour tortilla shells | 8 |
| ½ cup | pasta sauce (meatless) | 125 mL |
| 2 oz | goat cheese | 50 g |
| 2 oz | shredded part-skim Mozzarella cheese | 50 g |

1. Lightly spray peppers, zucchini and mushroom caps with olive oil flavored cooking spray. Season vegetables with rosemary and freshly ground pepper.
2. Grill vegetables on a non-stick grill pan or under the broiler in the oven. Set aside.
3. Place 2 tortilla shells flat on top of each other on a non-stick baking sheet. Spread with 2 tbsp/25 mL sauce.
3. Place a few grilled pepper strips, zucchini rounds and sliced mushroom caps on sauce.
4. Dot with ½ oz/15 g crumbled goat cheese and sprinkle with ½ oz/15 g shredded part-skim Mozzarella cheese.
5. Repeat procedure with remaining ingredients to make 4 pizzas in total.
6. Bake in a 350 F/180°C oven for 10 minutes or until cheese is melted and golden brown.

Makes 4 pizzas.

# Quiche and Tell

Your guests will want to know the secret ingredient in this light and delicious crustless quiche. You can tell them it's egg whites.

| | | |
|---|---|---|
| 1 tsp | canola oil | 5 mL |
| ½ each | red and yellow bell pepper, seeded and chopped | ½ each |
| 1 | small onion, chopped | 1 |
| ½ lb | mushrooms, sliced | 250 g |
| 1 | clove garlic, minced | 1 |
| 1 tbsp | fresh parsley, chopped | 15 mL |
| | salt, pepper (to taste) | |
| | cooking spray | |
| 8 | egg whites or 1 cup / 250 mL egg whites in a carton | 8 |
| 2 tsp | grated Parmesan cheese | 10 mL |

1. Cook peppers, onion, mushrooms and garlic in 1 tsp of oil on medium-high heat. Season with salt and pepper to taste.
2. Add parsley and continue to cook until vegetables are softened. Set aside.
3. Lightly beat egg whites in a large bowl. Add vegetables and stir to combine.
4. Spray a round glass pie dish with cooking spray. Add egg white/vegetable mixture. Sprinkle with Parmesan cheese.
4. Bake in a 350°F/180°C oven for 30 minutes or until quiche is puffed and golden brown.
5. Remove from oven and let stand 10 minutes before cutting and serving.

Makes 4 servings.

# *Festive Meatballs*

Serve these yummy turkey meatballs as a lighter alternative to cocktail weenies at your next party. Or enjoy them for a family supper with brown rice and a salad. They're sure to please.

| | | |
|---|---|---|
| 1 lb | lean ground turkey, | 500 g |
| 4 | egg whites or ½ cup/125 mL egg whites in a carton, lightly beaten | 4 |
| ½ cup | bread or cracker crumbs, or matzo meal | 125 mL |
| ½ tsp | garlic powder | 2 mL |
| ½ tsp | black pepper | 2 mL |
| ½ tsp | Worcestershire sauce | 2 mL |
| ½ tsp | salt (or to taste) | 2 mL |
| 1 | 28 oz / 796 mL can crushed tomatoes | 1 |
| 2 tbsp | ketchup | 25 mL |
| ½ cup | jellied cranberry sauce | 125 mL |
| 1 tbsp | balsamic vinegar | 15 mL |
| | black pepper | |

1. Combine first 7 ingredients.
2. Fill a large pot half full with water. Bring water to a boil.
3. With wet hands form small meatballs and gently place meatballs in boiling water. Simmer meatballs uncovered over medium-high heat. Skim off foam.
4. When meatballs are cooked and no longer pink, remove meatballs from water with a slotted spoon. Discard water, rinse out pot and replace meatballs in pot.
5. In a saucepan, combine crushed tomatoes, ketchup, cranberry sauce and vinegar. Heat until cranberry sauce dissolves.
6. Gently pour sauce over meatballs, season with black pepper, cover and simmer for 1 hour.

Makes 6 servings.

**The Lowdown**
(per serving)

| | |
|---|---|
| calories | 259 |
| fat | 8 g |
| carbohydrate | 27 g |
| protein | 19 g |

**Highlight**

You can use lean ground chicken, veal or beef in this recipe. The fat and calorie content will vary.

# Light and Easy Potato Latkes

**The Lowdown**
(per latke)

| | |
|---|---|
| calories | 35 |
| fat | 0 g |
| carbohydrate | 8 g |
| protein | 1 g |

These are great at Chanukah and all year round. They make a terrific side-dish served with fat-free sour cream or unsweetened applesauce.

| | | |
|---|---|---|
| 1 | onion, peeled and sliced | 1 |
| 2 | egg whites or ¼ cup/50 mL egg whites in a carton | 2 |
| 3 | large baking potatoes, peeled and cubed | 3 |
| 3 tbsp | all-purpose flour | 45 mL |
| ½ tsp | baking powder | 2 mL |
| ½ tsp | salt | 2 mL |
| ¼ tsp | pepper | 1 mL |
| | cooking spray | |

1. Place first 7 ingredients in a food processor fitted with the steel blade.
2. Process using pulses until potato is finely chopped.
3. Spray a large non-stick frying pan with cooking spray.
3. Over medium-high heat, spoon about 1 heaping tablespoon / 15 mL batter per latke onto pan.
4. Cook latkes for a few minutes on each side until browned. Repeat with remaining batter until all latkes are cooked.
5. Serve immediately or keep warm in a 300°F / 150°C oven.

Makes 24 latkes.

# "You Look Mahvellous" Matzo Pizza

Yes, you can enjoy pizza, even at Passover, just substitute a board of matzo for the traditional pizza crust. It tastes just like a thin-crust gourmet pizza. Mahvellous!

| | | |
|---|---|---|
| 1 | board matzo | 1 |
| ¼ cup | marinara sauce | 50 mL |
| ½ cup | green and red peppers strips, sliced mushrooms and onions | 125 mL |
| 1 oz | part-skim Mozzarella cheese, shredded cooking spray | 25 g |

1. Spray baking sheet with cooking spray.
2. Place matzo on baking sheet. Spread matzo with marinara sauce. Arrange peppers, mushrooms and onions over sauce and top with shredded cheese.
3. Bake in 375°F/190°C oven for about 10 minutes or until cheese is melted.

Makes 1 pizza.

**The Lowdown**
(per pizza)

| | |
|---|---|
| calories | 237 |
| fat | 6 g |
| carbohydrate | 33 g |
| protein | 13 g |

# Passover The Mushroom Farfel Kugel

This is a lightened up version of a traditional recipe. Your guests won't be able to pass it up.

**The Lowdown**
(per serving)

| | |
|---|---|
| calories | 130 |
| fat | 1 g |
| carbohydrate | 27 g |
| protein | 4 g |

| | | |
|---|---|---|
| 16 oz | matzo farfel | 500 g |
| 4 cups | defatted chicken broth | 1 L |
| | vegetable cooking spray | |
| 1 | Spanish onion, chopped | 1 |
| ½ lb | mushrooms, sliced | 250 g |
| ½ each | green and red pepper, seeded and chopped | ½ each |
| 1 | carrot, grated | 1 |
| 4 | egg whites or ½ cup egg whites in a carton, lightly beaten | 4 |
| ½ tsp each | salt, black pepper, garlic powder (or to taste) | 2 mL each |
| | cooking spray | |

1. In a large mixing bowl, combine matzo farfel and heated chicken broth. Set aside.
2. On medium high heat, cook onion in a little water in a large non-stick skillet sprayed with cooking spray. Add green pepper, carrot and mushrooms and continue to cook until vegetables are softened.
3. Combine softened vegetables with matzo farfel mixture. Add beaten egg whites, salt, pepper, and garlic powder, to taste.
4. Turn mixture into a 9 x 12-inch / 3.5 L glass baking dish sprayed with cooking spray.
5. Bake in a 350° F / 180° C for one hour or until golden brown.

Makes 16 servings.

# Luscious Fruit and Berry Compote

Serve this luscious compote when peaches and plums are in season. For an elegant dessert, spoon compote into cut-glass dessert bowls or big wine goblets. Crown with a small scoop of vanilla frozen yogurt.

| | | |
|---|---|---|
| 4 | peaches, pitted and sliced | 4 |
| 4 | red or purple plums, pitted and quartered | 4 |
| 4 | apricots, pitted and quartered | 4 |
| 1 pint | blueberries | 500 mL |
| 2 tbsp | sugar (or equivalent sweetener) | 25 mL |
| 1 cup | raspberries | 250 mL |

1. Combine peaches, plums, apricots and blueberries in a large glass casserole. Sprinkle with sugar or sweetener.
2. Bake in a 350°F/180°C oven for 35 minutes. Remove from oven and allow to cool.
3. Carefully fold in raspberries, cover casserole and refrigerate.

Makes 8 servings.

**The Lowdown**
(per serving)

| | |
|---|---|
| calories | 82 |
| fat | 0 g |
| carbohydrate | 20 g |
| protein | 1 g |

**Highlight**

If fresh apricots are unavailable, leave them out. Just use more peaches or plums. Any combination will work.

# *Heavenly Chocolate Meringues*

Sweet as a kiss and light as air, these meringues are a heavenly treat. Perfect for Valentine's Day and all year round to show how much you care.

| | | |
|---|---|---|
| 1 cup | granulated sugar | 250 mL |
| 2 tbsp | unsweetened cocoa | 25 mL |
| 4 | egg whites or ½ cup egg whites in a carton, at room temperature | 4 |
| ¼ tsp | cream of tartar | 1 mL |
| ½ tsp | vanilla | 2 mL |
| ¼ cup | mini-chocolate chips | 50 mL |

1. Sift together the sugar and cocoa. Set aside.
2. Beat together the egg whites, vanilla and cream of tartar at high speed until they form stiff peaks.
3. Carefully fold in the sugar/cocoa mixture and the chocolate chips.
4. Drop by rounded teaspoons onto a baking tray lined with parchment or wax paper.
5. Bake in a 250°F/120°C oven for 1½ to 2 hours or until meringues are crispy. For extra crispy meringues, turn the oven off at the end of baking and leave meringues in the oven for one hour more.

Makes 48 meringues.

# Cola Baked Apples

Serve warm or chilled, topped with a dollop of fat-free vanilla yogurt.

| | | |
|---|---|---|
| 4 | medium-sized Spy or cooking apples, washed and cored | 4 |
| 2 tsp | sugar or equivalent sweetener | 10 mL |
| 1 tsp | cinnamon | 5 mL |
| 1 cup | sugar-free cola | 250 mL |

1. Place apples in an 8-inch / 2 L baking pan. Pierce apple skins in several places with a fork.
2. Sprinkle sugar and cinnamon into center of each apple.
3. Pour sugar-free cola into bottom of baking pan.
4. Bake in a 375°F / 190°C oven for 45 minutes or until apples are soft. Baste with cola several times while apples are baking.

Makes 4 servings.

**The Lowdown**
(per serving)

| | |
|---|---|
| calories | 87 |
| fat | 0 g |
| carbohydrate | 22 g |
| protein | 0 g |

**Highlight**

This recipe can be cooked in the microwave. Cover apples and cook on High for 5-7 minutes or until apples are soft. Baste with cola half way through the cooking time.

# Apple Raisin Crisp With A-peel

This dish is perfect any time you want a real treat. To save time and to boost fiber content, you don't have to peel the apples. For variety, you can use a combination of apples and pears in this recipe.

| 6 | medium-sized Spartan or Spy apples washed, cored, sliced, peeled or unpeeled | 6 |
|---|---|---|
| 1 tsp | cinnamon | 5 mL |
| | cooking spray | |
| 2 tbsp | brown sugar or equivalent sweetener | 25 mL |
| 1 cup | bran cereal with raisins | 250 mL |
| 1 tsp | non-hydrogenated margarine | 5 mL |

1. Toss apple slices with cinnamon.
2. Place apple slices in an 8-inch / 2 L baking dish sprayed with cooking spray.
3. Top apples with brown sugar and cereal. Dot with margarine.
4. Cover with foil and bake in a 375° F / 190° C oven for 45 minutes or until fruit is cooked. Uncover and bake for 5 minutes more.

Makes 6 servings.

# PART 3

# *Personal Journal*

239

A S YOU BEGIN YOUR JOURNEY toward living life in a healthy way, you'll need to do some planning to make sure you reach your destination of eating well, being active and feeling good about yourself, once and for all. You'll need strategies for making the changes that will ensure your success. The self-awareness tools in Part 3 are designed to help you achieve your goals.

# Personal Journal

# Eating Awareness Quiz

Score _____ /10

Check off each statement that applies to you. Count the number of checks and score yourself out of 10. The higher the score, the more changes you'll need to make.

☐ 1. I usually skip breakfast.

☐ 2. I use terms like good, bad, control and cheat when it comes to food.

☐ 3. I eat in places other than the kitchen or dining-room.

☐ 4. I reward myself with food.

☐ 5. I eat standing up, while I'm preparing food or doing other things.

☐ 6. I find it hard to resist tempting food, especially in a social situation.

☐ 7. I eat few, if any vegetables.

☐ 8. I eat when I'm upset, tired or bored.

☐ 9. When I start eating, sometimes I can't stop.

☐ 10. I drink a cup or two of water daily.

# Setting Goals

To help you set goals for yourself, complete the following sentences.

1. My personal healthy eating and lifestyle goals are

_____

_____

_____

2. So far I've been able to accomplish the following

_____

_____

_____

3. The challenges that I still face are

_____

_____

_____

4. My personal strengths are

_____

_____

_____

5. I can use these strengths to achieve my goals by

_____

_____

_____

# Breakfast for Champions

Start your day with a healthy breakfast and the rest of the day will follow. Your breakfast doesn't have to be fancy or be eaten at the crack of dawn. It should include three of the four food groups and be consumed sometime before lunch. Doing this quiz will help.

## Complete the following statements.

1. In the past week, I have eaten breakfast _____ times.

2. When I eat breakfast I feel _____

3. When I don't eat breakfast, I feel _____

4. I sometimes skip breakfast because _____

5. If I could eat anything for breakfast it would be _____

6. I could have a similar but lighter breakfast by choosing _____

_____

7. Three of the four food groups which I've included in my breakfast are

_____

8. For a healthy breakfast on the weekend when I have more time, I will treat myself to

_____

# Be a Trans Fat Detective

Look at the label on a processed food that you have in your kitchen. If the fat information is given, calculate the hidden fat which likely contains trans fat.

Sample Food:_____

Total Fat (per serving) _____ g

    Polyunsaturated fat _____ g

    Monounsaturated fat _____ g

    Saturated fat _____ g

    Total (P+M+S) _____ g

Total Fat (per serving) - Total (P+M+S) = Unidentified Fat

_____ g – _____ g = _____ g

The amount of potentially cholesterol-raising fat is

_____ g (Saturated fat) + _____ g (Unidentified fat) = _____ g.

## Figuring the Fat

Now calculate the percentage of calories coming from fat in your sample food.

Fat (per serving)_____ g x 9 calories per gram = _____ calories from fat.

_____ calories from fat divided by _____ calories per serving

= _____ x 100% = _____ % calories coming from fat.

## Conclusion

The amount of potentially cholesterol-raising fat is _____ g.

The percentage of calories coming from fat is _____%.

I will choose this food _____ (often, sometimes, infrequently).

# Water Works Quiz

Complete these sentences.

1. At the present time, I drink about _____ cups of water per day.

2. I drink _____ cups of regular or decaf tea, coffee and soft drinks.

3. I eat salad _____ times per week.

4. I have soup _____ times per week.

5. I drink a cup of juice _____ times per week.

6. I estimate that I consume about _____ cups of fluid per day.

7. I need to increase my intake by _____ cups per day.

8. I can do this by

_____

_____

_____

_____

9. I will start increasing my fluids today by

_____

_____

_____

_____

_____

# The Lighter Weigh

When you're ready, follow these steps to determine your healthy weight goal:

1. calculate your BMI to determine if your weight is in the healthy range
2. record your lowest adult weight and how long you maintained this weight
3. calculate your Waist to Hip Ratio (WHR) to determine if you are an apple or a pear, by dividing your waist by your hip measurement
4. review your family tree for possible weight trends
5. assess your weight as it affects your feeling of well-being
6. fine-tune your healthy weight goal as you go along

## 1. Body Mass Index

My current weight is _____ kg.* My current height is _____ cm.**

My current height is _____ meters.*** My height in meters squared is _____.

To determine your BMI, divide your weight in kilograms by your height in meters squared.

_____ kg divided by _____ meters squared = _____ BMI.

BMI <20 underweight, 20-25 healthy weight, 25-27 caution,****
>27 above a healthy weight.

My BMI is in the _____ range.

## 2. Personal Weight History

My lowest adult weight is _____ kg.

My highest adult weight is _____ kg.

My lowest adult weight that I was able to maintain for at least 2 years is_____ kg.

---

\*      to convert from pounds to kilograms, divide by 2.2
\*\*     to convert from inches to centimeters, multiply by 2.54
\*\*\*    to convert from centimeters to meters, divide by 100
\*\*\*\*   a BMI of 25–29 is considered overweight by the World Health Organization

### 3. Waist to Hip Ratio (WHR)

My waist measurement is _____ cm.

My hip measurement is _____ cm.

My waist divided by my hip measurement is

_____ cm divided by _____ cm = _____.

My WHR is _____ .

_____ I am an "apple" (WHR female >0.8, male >1.0)

_____ I am a "pear" (WHR female < 0.8, male <1.0).

### 4. Family History

A noticeable weight trend in my family is _____
(Underweight, average weight, overweight, there doesn't appear to be a trend)

### 5. Medical History

Medical conditions which my doctor suggested could be improved with weight reduction are

_____

(High blood pressure, high cholesterol, type 2 diabetes, other).

### 6. How I Feel

At my present weight, I feel _____
(Tired, energetic, the way I've always felt, I could feel better, other).

### My Realistic Healthy Weight Goal is _____

(Be sure to reassess this goal from time to time to make sure that it stays realistic for you.)

# Feel Good Rewards

Reward yourself as you start achieving your goals. Important milestones should be recognized. Going for a whole day without multiples, choosing a lighter meal at your favorite restaurant or reaching your first mini-weight goal are all reasons to celebrate. The following is a suggested list of non-food rewards. Add your choices below.

## Non-food Rewards

1. a long soak in a bubble bath
2. a massage
3. a manicure
4. a phone call to a special friend
5. a shoe shine
6. a romance novel
7. a subscription to a magazine
8. a new workout outfit
9. a pedicure
10. a new shade of lipstick
11. a new hairstyle
12. a beauty makeover
13. a new article of clothing
14. theater tickets for you and a friend
15. a walk in the park
16. a new CD
17. a membership at a gym
18. a new scarf
19. a new belt
20. a joke book

Your choices

1. _____
2. _____
3. _____
4. _____
5. _____
6. _____
7. _____
8. _____
9. _____
10. _____

# *Are you a Natural?*

You may already have some "natural" healthy lifestye habits. Take this quiz to find out.

Read each statement. Answer Y (yes) or N (no).

☐ 1. I always eat breakfast.

☐ 2. I eat when I'm hungry and stop when I'm full.

☐ 3. I eat more of my food earlier in the day when my body needs it.

☐ 4. I can handle multiples.

☐ 5. I combine regular physical activity with healthy eating.

☐ 6. I laugh every day as often as I can.

☐ 7. I try not to wear expandable waistbands.

☐ 8. I seldom eat while I'm doing other things.

☐ 9. I enjoy fruit for dessert.

☐ 10. I balance higher fat foods with lighter choices.

Total the number of times you answered Y (yes). These are your healthy habits. The number of healthy habits I have is _____

Total the number of times you answered N (no). These are the habits that still need work. The number of healthy habits that still need work are _____

The habit which I will start working on today is _____

A healthy habit which I possess not mentioned above is

_____

# Light Stuff Shopping List

**Fresh Vegetables and Vegetarian Products**

- [ ] salad greens (fresh or bagged)
- [ ] cucumber
- [ ] tomatoes
- [ ] peppers
- [ ] fresh herbs (parsley, basil, rosemary, cilantro, thyme, oregano, dill)
- [ ] potatoes
- [ ] garlic
- [ ] broccoli
- [ ] cauliflower
- [ ] carrots
- [ ] cabbage (white, red)
- [ ] onions
- [ ] celery
- [ ] zucchini
- [ ] green beans
- [ ] eggplant
- [ ] bean sprouts
- [ ] mushrooms
- [ ] tofu

- [ ] soy veggie slices
- [ ] soy veggie ground "beef"
- [ ] dehydrated soy protein
- [ ] other _____
  _____
  _____

**Fresh Fruit**

- [ ] bananas
- [ ] apples
- [ ] oranges, orange juice
- [ ] pears
- [ ] melon (cantaloupe or honeydew)
- [ ] pineapple (golden or regular)
- [ ] berries (strawberries, blueberries, raspberries)
- [ ] kiwi
- [ ] mango
- [ ] lemon, lime
- [ ] dried fruit (raisins, prunes, apricots, cranberries)
- [ ] other _____
  _____

## Dairy Delights

- ☐ skim milk (regular or lactose-reduced)
- ☐ fat-free yogurt
- ☐ 1% cottage cheese
- ☐ part-skim Mozzarella cheese
- ☐ low-fat or fat-free cheese slices
- ☐ low-fat feta cheese
- ☐ grated Parmesan cheese
- ☐ fat-free sour cream
- ☐ egg whites in a carton
- ☐ low-fat soy drink
- ☐ other _____
  _____

## Meat of the Matter

- ☐ extra-lean ground beef, veal, chicken, turkey
- ☐ stewing cubes of lean beef or veal
- ☐ boneless, skinless chicken breasts
- ☐ chicken carcass
- ☐ turkey breast, thighs, wings
- ☐ fish fillets (sole, halibut, haddock, cod)
- ☐ other _____
  _____

## Bread Basket

- ☐ whole grain sliced bread
- ☐ whole wheat pita
- ☐ whole grain bagels (2 oz/50 g size)
- ☐ whole wheat English muffins
- ☐ bread crumbs
- ☐ other _____
  _____

## Healthy Fats

- ☐ olive oil
- ☐ canola oil
- ☐ sunflower oil
- ☐ cooking spray (regular, olive oil, butter flavor)
- ☐ sesame oil
- ☐ other _____
  _____

## Condiments, Spices, Dried Herbs

- ☐ Dijon mustard
- ☐ honey mustard
- ☐ ketchup
- ☐ balsamic vinegar
- ☐ red wine vinegar

- [ ] seasoned rice vinegar
- [ ] low-sodium soy sauce
- [ ] low-fat Italian salad dressing
- [ ] ultra-light mayonnaise
- [ ] salsa
- [ ] apple butter
- [ ] fruit spread
- [ ] tahini or peanut butter
- [ ] black pepper
- [ ] dried herbs (basil, oregano, parsley, rosemary, thyme, tarragon)
- [ ] garlic powder
- [ ] cinnamon
- [ ] cumin
- [ ] capers
- [ ] dried onion flakes
- [ ] hot pepper sauce
- [ ] other _____

_____

## Cereal

- [ ] cold unsweetened cereal
- [ ] oatmeal
- [ ] instant oatmeal
- [ ] instant cream of wheat

- [ ] natural bran
- [ ] wheat germ
- [ ] cornflake crumbs
- [ ] other _____

_____

## Crackers, Cookies, Snack Foods

- [ ] baked chips
- [ ] pretzels
- [ ] microwave popcorn
- [ ] rice cakes
- [ ] melba toast
- [ ] arrowroot biscuits
- [ ] graham wafers
- [ ] Swedish flatbread
- [ ] other _____

_____

## Frozen Foods

- [ ] frozen vegetables (California, Italian, Oriental)
- [ ] frozen fish fillets
- [ ] frozen skinless boneless chicken breasts
- [ ] frozen yogurt bars

- [ ] ice milk bars
- [ ] other _____
  _____

## Canned Goods

- [ ] crushed tomatoes
- [ ] stewed tomatoes
- [ ] water-packed tuna
- [ ] salmon
- [ ] chickpeas
- [ ] kidney beans
- [ ] black beans
- [ ] lentils
- [ ] corn niblets
- [ ] sliced water chestnuts
- [ ] baby corn
- [ ] mandarin orange segments
- [ ] fat-free chicken broth
- [ ] other _____
  _____

## Dry Goods

- [ ] pasta
- [ ] rice (brown, white, basmati, wild)

- [ ] couscous
- [ ] kasha
- [ ] barley
- [ ] other _____
  _____

## 12. Baking Needs

- [ ] whole wheat flour
- [ ] all-purpose flour
- [ ] baking powder
- [ ] baking soda
- [ ] vanilla
- [ ] unsweetened applesauce
- [ ] sugar
- [ ] sweetener
- [ ] icing sugar
- [ ] mini-chocolate chips
- [ ] other _____
  _____

## Soft Drinks, Beverages, Juices

- [ ] sugar-free soft drinks
- [ ] mineral or bottled water
- [ ] herbal tea

- ☐ decaf tea
- ☐ decaf coffee
- ☐ tomato juice
- ☐ vegetable juice cocktail

- ☐ cranberry juice cocktail
- ☐ other _____

_____

_____

# Social-Lighting

Healthy eating can be a real challenge when you're eating out. With a few well-planned strategies, you can handle even the toughest situations with ease.

Describe a challenging eating out situation for you. _____
_____
_____

How did you handle it? _____
_____
_____

What lighter food choices were you able to make? _____
_____
_____

How do you feel about the way you handled this situation? _____
_____
_____

What, if anything, would you do differently next time? _____
_____
_____

How did you feel when the meal was over? _____
_____
_____

What did you learn from this eating out experience? _____
_____
_____

# Workout Personality Profile

Circle (A) or (B). There are no right or wrong answers.

1. I like to work out (A) alone or (B) in a class.
2. I like to wear (A) a workout outfit or (B) a baggy T-shirt suits me just fine.
3. I like (A) the challenge of a game or (B) games are too stressful for me.
4. I like to (A) repeat the same activities or (B) I get bored easily.

Compare your answers to the workout personality profiles in Chapter 9 and answer the following questions.

My workout type is _____

_____

_____

The activities suited to my type are _____

_____

_____

What I can realistically start doing now is _____

_____

_____

What I plan to start doing soon is _____

_____

_____

I can live actively every day by _____

_____

_____

_____

# Lighten Up Your Eating Plan

In the left-hand column, record what you eat in one day. In the right-hand column, write down some choices you can make to lighten up, the way we did in Chapter 10.

## What I Usually Eat

Breakfast

_____

_____

_____

Lunch

_____

_____

_____

Snack

_____

_____

Dinner

_____

_____

_____

_____

_____

Snack

_____

_____

_____

## How I Can Lighten Up

Breakfast

_____

_____

_____

Lunch

_____

_____

_____

Snack

_____

_____

Dinner

_____

_____

_____

_____

Snack

_____

_____

_____

# *Trigger Happy*

The most appropriate cue or "trigger" for eating is hunger. There are, however, many other cues that can stimulate you to eat. Identifying these triggers will help you to eat when you are truly hungry. Then you'll be "trigger happy".

An inappropriate trigger for eating can be a person, a place, an activity, an emotion, a time of day, or one of your senses. For example, being with someone with whom you usually overeat may be a trigger to eat, even when you're not hungry. Being in a place like the kitchen or the den, or doing an activity like watching TV or seeing a movie can also be triggers. A time of day like four o'clock in the afternoon can be a trigger, especially if it's been a snacking time for you. Emotions like anger, frustration or worry are also triggers for some people, as are the smell or sight of a favorite food. Complete this quiz to help you identify your personal triggers.

Describe an eating situation in which the trigger to eat was something other than hunger.

_____

_____

_____

Let's see if you can identify the triggers.

1. Who was with you? _____

2. Where were you? _____

3. What were you doing? _____

_____

4. What time of day was it? _____

5. How were you feeling? _____

6. Were any of your senses involved? _____

_____

Think about your answers. What conclusions can you draw about the triggers that played a role in this situation.

1. The following triggers played a role in my eating

_____

_____

_____

_____

2. How can you use what you have learned to handle a similar situation in the future?

_____

_____

_____

_____

3. Make a list of your personal triggers. Beside each one, record how you can handle or avoid this trigger.

| Trigger | How to Handle or Avoid |
|---|---|
| _____ | _____ |
| _____ | _____ |
| _____ | _____ |
| _____ | _____ |
| _____ | _____ |
| _____ | _____ |
| _____ | _____ |

# Daily Affirmations

To help you reach your healthy lifestyle goals, it is important to remind yourself of all the good things that you are doing for yourself. Do this warm-up daily to help you appreciate how far you've come and stay focused on where you're going. After you've completed your answers, read or say them aloud to yourself. Reread them anytime you need a boost. You'll see how good you'll feel.

1. My goals are _____

   _____

   _____

2. So far I have accomplished _____

   _____

   _____

   _____

3. Three things in my life that I am grateful for today are

   _____

   _____

   _____

4. Today I will _____

   _____

   _____

5. I feel _____

   _____

   _____

# Healthy Eating Plan

In the blank spaces provided, indicate the number of servings per day you will be aiming for. You can use your national food guide or the sample menus in Chapter 10 as a guide.

Always consult your doctor before making changes to your food and activity habits. You may want to discuss this plan with your doctor and/or dietitian before you proceed.

## My Healthy Eating Plan
### Number of Servings per Day

_____ Grains and Starches     _____ Milk Products

_____ Vegetables              _____ Meats and Alternatives

_____ Fruits                  _____ Fats and Oils

## Daily Food and Activity Diary

Record everything you eat and drink in one day, the time you eat, the type of food and beverages, and the serving size. Also indicate how much water you have consumed and what type of activities you have engaged in and for how long.

Total your intake of food and beverages in the space provided and compare it to your healthy eating plan that you have chosen for yourself.

Today is _____

Breakfast (time: _____ )

_____

_____

_____

Lunch (time: _____ )

_____

_____

_____

_____

Snack (time: _____ )

_____

Dinner (time: _____ )

_____

_____

_____

_____

Snack (time: _____ )

_____

**Activity type** _____ **Time spent** _____

**Cups of water** ☐ ☐ ☐ ☐ ☐ ☐ ☐ ☐

### Daily Totals

_____ Grains and Starches     _____ Milk Products

_____ Vegetables     _____ Meats and Alts

_____ Fruits     _____ Fats and Oils

# Personal Journal

You may find it helpful to keep a journal to write down your thoughts and feelings, either on a daily basis or from time to time. Use this and the following pages in whatever way suits you. Personal Journal is your special place.

_____

_____

_____

_____

_____

_____

_____

_____

_____

_____

_____

_____

_____

_____

_____

_____

_____

# Personal Journal

_____

_____

_____

_____

_____

_____

_____

_____

_____

_____

_____

_____

_____

_____

_____

_____

_____

_____

_____

_____

_____

# Personal Journal

# Subject Index

# Recipe Index